YOGA FOR T

Shows how the philosophy and practice of this ancient
tradition can improve the quality of your life.

YOGA
—FOR THE—
DISABLED

A Practical Self-Help Guide to a Happier Healthier Life

by

Howard Kent

SUNRISE PUBLICATIONS
Ickwell Bury, Biggleswade SG18 9EF

First published 1985
Reprinted 1996

British Library Cataloguing in Publication Data

Kent, Howard
    Yoga for the disabled: a practical self-help
    guide to a happier healthier life.
    1. Yoga. Hatha. 2. Physical education for
    handicapped persons
    I. Title
    613.7'046'0880816   RA781.7

    ISBN 0-7225-0902-2

Printed and bound in Great Britain
by Stanley L. Hunt (Printers) Ltd, Midland Road, Rushden, Northants

CONTENTS

INTRODUCTION

It is right to say something about the background upon which this book is written. My interest in yoga dates back to the late 1930s, but my realization that yoga is central to fighting the problems of disablement is much more recent.

In 1970 I produced a television series called *Yoga for Health*. This introduced the subject to millions of people in Britain and many other countries. Among the many thousands of letters I received, while the series was being screened, was one from a senior physiotherapist in Scotland. She said she had become interested in yoga and felt that it would provide greater benefits for those with multiple sclerosis than normal physiotherapy. With the support of her local branch of the MS Society she began a small weekly group and monitored their progress very carefully, taking muscle tests and series of photographs. Within three months she was convinced of the rightness of her belief. Although she had to give up the group, it is still running successfully.

This development coincided with a growing realization of the value of yoga in all forms of chronic ill-health. The Multiple Sclerosis Society showed interest from the beginning and other small groups were started. At this time the small organization I had formed employed a clinical psychologist to organize this work and it extended into many other areas of disablement.

The organization became a registered charity, the Yoga for Health Foundation, and in 1978, without money but with plenty of faith, we took a lease on a large and beautiful property in Bedfordshire to run as a residential centre. In the seven years which have ensued, Ickwell Bury has received thousands of guests with all kinds of disabling conditions and, increasingly, they have come from almost all parts of the world. During this period the realization of what yoga has to offer has grown considerably and the results have been most encouraging.

I can claim no specialist medical knowledge: this is neither an apology nor a boast. For a practitioner of yoga to take an active interest in disablement does demand study and common sense but, as will be seen from the ensuing pages, yoga is not a medical approach in the normal sense of the word; it is an understanding of how we can marshal the strength of both body and mind to combat our problems. No difficulty is purely physical, nor is it purely a matter of the mind: all are psychophysical . . . a complex integration of what is generally called the psyche and of the body itself.

In recent years I have, however, benefited immensely from the practical guidance and support of members of the medical profession, four of whom I would like to thank here. They are Professor A. Andreasen, who has become consultant in remedial medicine to us at our Centre and whose immense knowledge, wisdom and good spirits have inspired us greatly; Dr David Clark, a distinguished psychiatrist, whose background has been very valuable; Dr Barbara Brosnan, whose example in the yoga running of a home for the disabled in London, has been most inspiring; and Dr Ann Woolley-Hart, a research doctor, who has helped greatly in assessing the areas in which methods of research are helpful and those in which they are merely an encumbrance.

Those who have worked at Ickwell Bury have also contributed greatly to my own growth and experience, but above all I must thank the guests, many of them with severe physical problems, who have shown me strength and courage and have offered me warmth and friendship.

This book is intended for the person with physical disablement; I hope, too, it will be useful to many others, including yoga teachers, medical practitioners and paramedicals, who have a special interest. I am always happy to try to help and answer questions about yoga and its value.

HOWARD KENT,
Yoga for Health Foundation,
Ickwell Bury, Northill,
Biggleswade, Bedfordshire.

1.

THE CONCEPT OF YOGA

The dilemma of the human being is encapsulated in that sad phrase, 'I wish I . . .' We long for changes, mental and physical, feel we cannot achieve them and, all too often, nurse the resulting sense of frustration.

What changes *can* we bring about in our lives? What actual limits are there to our capacities? We all have the feeling that we can achieve far more than we think possible if only we can see how. This is a book about physical disablement; how we oppose it where we can; how we live with it where opposition is useless.

It is not as yet widely apparent, but a revolution is currently taking place in medical thought. Recently, a group of doctors met in conference and agreed that, at least in theory, there is no illness which the human body cannot overcome. If this growing feeling is right, out of the window go such words as 'incurable' and 'degenerative': instead, we declare that we have misunderstood the whole concept of ill-health. While it is a word often misused, such views come under the omnibus heading of 'holistic', which has now joined 'ecological' as a signpost of a new understanding of the life-process. 'Holistic' signifies the two 'I's' which struggle in the 'I wish I . . .' concept: the apparent Jekyll and Hyde of human existence, summed up by Lady Macbeth as, 'Letting ''I dare not'' wait upon ''I would'' . . .'

It is important to keep in the forefront of our mind the fact that each one of us with the good fortune to be born with normally functioning limbs has already performed a miracle — quite unaided. During the first months of our life we were little more than bundles, sometimes inert, sometimes kicking and screaming. We lay, because we could do no other; if we were made to stand up, we fell down. Yet not long after, we were toddling, then walking; our arms began to hold things and direct things. We had achieved harmonious movement and the co-ordination of our limbs. How did this miracle come about? We had no lectures on the subject. No one offered us a course in walking. Mother did not pop a 'Walk in Easy Lessons' book in our hands. The first 'I' knew it had to do it and had no means of expressing doubt — for we had not learned language and knew nothing of 'I can't'. Imagine us now, with words, thoughts and conditioning at our command, called upon to perform a corresponding feat to that of walking. 'No way,' we would shout. 'Impossible,' the professionals would agree. So we would sit behind the walls of the prison we had made for ourselves.

What *can* the human being achieve?

The simple answer is that we do not know. But the simple challenge is to find out. I have watched people with a definitive problem, such as spina bifida, work on themselves with a cheery smile and calm determination over a period of years. They still had spina bifida, but what they could achieve physically and what they could enjoy in life were both enormously enhanced. Almost certainly their life expectancy was enhanced also. I have also watched people with an amorphous problem, such as multiple sclerosis, work on themselves with the same cheery smile and calm determination. During a period of years they have slowly but surely overcome physical handicaps and also have become more truly happy. Occasionally, of course, there are dramatic improvements, even permanent remissions, but these are likely to prove the exception — however welcome an exception — and we do best to consider the less spectacular, steady improvement.

With the 'New Age' medical doctors I would say that this is what happens when a human being begins to realize his or her true capacity and can apply this realization quietly and with a steady diminution of tension. And is not the most exciting thing in life that which we have achieved for ourselves? There is no greater satisfaction. The big question is how do we do it? For the answer we must go back to the baby. The baby did not know the word 'How?' He did not waste time intellectualizing. Something inside stirred him and he simply got on with the job. Now we are dominated by words, by thoughts, by memories and by suggestions which we cannot simply block out. So we must make use of them: clear, logical thought must bring us back to the pure intuition which spurred us on in our infancy. This is where yoga comes in.

What is yoga?
What *is* yoga? It is neither standing on one's head nor contemplating one's navel. It is a word from the ancient Eastern classical language, Sanskrit. It means 'integration' or 'union' and is a declaration that we are all of us an integral part of the whole force of life. Increasingly, we can realize that this is not a metaphysical statement, it is a scientific one. Such a view is integral to spiritual teachings. Jesus Christ is said to have declared, 'The Kingdom of God is within you'. The Gospel of St. Thomas, while not included in the books of the Bible, goes even further and says that Christ declared God's Kingdom is both within and without — in other words it is all-pervasive. Ancient Eastern spiritual wisdom answers the question, 'Who am I?' by declaring, 'I am That' — That representing the universal force, or God, or whatever term you care to use. Great thinkers throughout the ages have expressed similar ideas in different ways. To put it simply, yoga declares that we are not alone, not isolated.

In our society life is based on a series of collectives. The first, and fundamental, is that of the family. The natural family unit is one in which the members feel strengthened and more secure by being a part of the family. Broadening out a little, we have a pride in — and feel we can relax in — our neighbourhood, our parish, our part of the world, our country. Presumably, if we do discover some equivalent of little green men from Mars, we will also develop a world identity to help us ward off the unknown. Through yoga, the concept of union, we say that there are no limitations to these feelings of community. They all express aspects of the universal linking; we are all part of the same great force. What has this to do with health and disablement? The answer is everything.

Our understanding of life

Our whole life depends upon our *idea* of life. If we are fundamentally insecure, this insecurity will show itself day by day in all our actions. Likewise a true sense of security, of belonging, will promote harmony and stability. Feelings of insecurity quickly promote feelings of guilt, often with disastrous effect. Here are three examples, all of people with multiple sclerosis. When Stanley was eight years old, he was running across the road with a friend named Johnny. A car came round a bend, knocked Johnny down and killed him. Stanley was so terrified that he ran off and never told anyone of the incident. So great was his guilt that he hid it from his conscious mind. Many years later, when he was a disabled man in his fifties, he was regressed by a hypnotherapist and recalled the incident. As a result he had a period of sobbing and then felt much better. Paul was a capable aqua-diver. A young man asked Paul to teach him the skill. Paul took him out in shallow water and then asked him to follow round to the other side of the bay. The young man disappeared. When the body was found, twenty-four hours later, it was discovered that he had foolishly eaten a meal shortly before entering the water. As a result he had vomited under water and suffocated himself. The parents did not blame Paul, but he blamed himself and could not get guilt for the incident out of his system. Kate was walking along a road as a child when a man coming towards her dropped down with a heart attack. Terrified, Kate ran off instead of trying to get help. All three now have multiple sclerosis; all three have it *only* in the legs.

It is not suggested, of course, that the MS was necessarily the result of the guilt feelings, but clearly the mind directed the disease into the part of the body about which they felt guilty. Paul, in fact, declared, 'I have often wanted to go round to that fellow's parents and say to them, "Look what's happened to me, now." '

A feeling of unity with life would not make us unconcerned in such circumstances, on the contrary, but the emotion would not be the crucifying one of guilt. Here is one more example. A man came to our yoga Residential Centre, quite unheralded, suffering from an appalling chest condition. He wheezed so much that he could hardly walk. It took two people to help him up to a first-floor bedroom. He was a business man of around fifty years old. It seemed that he had always had a troublesome chest, but nothing of any concern. Now his doctors told him that his only chance was to retire — almost a sentence of early death to such a man. Then I discovered that he was consumed with hatred. An associate had brought a court case against him and won. He swore he was framed. His entire life was spent plotting his revenge — and a mildly weak chest had changed into a killer condition. This man had tried doctors and clinics to no avail. But four weeks later he left our Centre running down the stairs with a suitcase in each hand, declaring that he must have left something out as they felt too light. Breathing training had helped him tremendously but the root of the change came from a new understanding of life itself, for hatred can only come from a feeling of fear and isolation.

This is not to suggest that we all have to keep searching back over the past to try to discover the root of our troubles. A few cases are obvious, but the majority are far more complex. The obvious ones simply help to underline the basis of our contention. We must, however, begin with acceptance. Whether or not we can see the 'hang-up' which is holding us back, so long as it remains, just so long is our power of opposition severely diminished. Medical research into that area of unrelieved tension which we now call stress has shown that the key emotion is resentment. In reality this is a portmanteau word incorporating frustration, anger, fear. The key is non-acceptance; the worm beneath the skin. Even when pushed to the back of the mind, or into the subconscious, such emotions are constantly subtly influencing physiological reaction throughout the body.

Why did it happen to me?
In disabling diseases and accidents, the repeatedly-asked
and quite unanswerable question is, 'Why did it happen to
me?' From observation of some thousands of people in
such circumstances, I would say that those who harbour
such a resentment — and its near-neighbours — never
show signs of combating their difficulties. Joyless and
enervated, they sink, perhaps slowly at first, but soon at
an ever-accelerating speed. Where you find people coping
with their disability, even slowly reversing it, you always
find an equable and accepting temperament. Acceptance
does not mean 'lying down under': it means accepting this
is the position, here and now, considering what is to be
done about it quietly and calmly. On such a basis, such
decisions can be implemented without undue strain.

Yoga straddles the mystical and the scientific. Where it is
appropriate to test the circumstances of yoga by scientific
means, it emerges triumphantly. To be a mystic is by no
means to deny science. One of the greatest mystics of our
century was Albert Einstein, also the most brilliant
scientific brain. Einstein wrote: 'What is the meaning of
human life, or of organic life altogether? To answer this
question at all implies a religion. Is there any sense then,
you ask, in putting it? I answer, the man who regards his
own life and that of his fellow creatures as meaningless is
not merely unfortunate but almost disqualified for life.'
Einstein did not purport to be able to discover or explain
that meaning — even the scientist's equations could not
help him here. The important thing is to realize that there
is a meaning and we are integrally involved in that
meaning.

If there is a meaning, it follows that our encapsulation in
a body is a part of that meaning and so the relationship
between 'us' and our body is central. The body is not
merely God's sick joke, a cage in which we are trapped for
a variable number of years. There would appear to be only
one alternative: if it is not there to trap 'us' — then
controlling it is a process in 'our' development.

First, though, what is this 'us'? The word used down the
ages is 'soul' and this was perhaps best defined by that
remarkable man of understanding, Carl Jung, who gave it

the name of *anima* in man and *animus* in woman. The soul, declared Jung, is a psychological reality. While, in our use of the word, it is unconscious, it is the basis of our conscious lives. In Jung's own phrase, the soul is 'both receiver and transmitter'. If, in our 'scientific age', such ideas seem far-fetched, in fact, the exact opposite is the case. The scientific realization of the amazing and wonderful complexity of matter, a complexity which is at the same time a unity, makes the step to accepting a soul, described in these terms, a very small one. There is, then, an essential 'us', lying behind and capable of directing the physical us. In Einstein's phrase, 'the meaning of life' would seem to be the growing control of the physical us by that soul, not as a selfish and ego-bound process but as part of the drive towards harmony.

The power of the yogis
How does yoga assist us in this process? Let us begin with one example. About three years ago, teams of doctors from the American Army Medical School and Harvard Medical School set out for India to investigate the claims of yogis that they could change their own body temperatures. For many years the medical view in the West has been that we can have little or no control over autonomic processes of the body. Skin temperature is obviously one of these processes. Thousands of messages from the skin relay information about the external temperature and feelings of comfort or discomfort are changed into signals of warm or cold. The body reacts automatically to such signals. This, then, we can say is reality, because it is my reaction to external conditions. The yogi, however, says that to a great degree reality lies not in the body but in the mind.

Conducting medical tests, the doctors investigating the claims found that the yogis concerned could indeed actually change the temperature on the skin of their bodies, in less than one hour, by as much as 15°F. They could do this either to the whole body or pre-selected parts of the body but nothing else about the body was affected. So the yogis had made their own reality and the body had responded. The mind was more powerful than the elements. We have only to imagine the difference between a chilly day with a temperature of 58°F and a warm summer's day with the temperature around 72°F to see the amazing change which the mind can bring about on the body. The type of doctor who believes that human beings are trapped in their bodies, unless they can be relieved by some wonder treatment offered by the physician, should study this investigation — and many other similar ones.

It is still possible to protest that the antics of a group of saffron-robed holy men in the Himalayas have very little relevance to us in the West. True, the background and disciplines of such people may seem alien to us but the most detailed possible investigation will reveal no physiological or mental difference. In fact, experiments conducted by volunteers at the Menninger Institute in America have shown that, rightly directed, we, too, can begin to produce the same results. It is only a matter of practice and understanding.

What was the process used by these yogis? It was amazingly simple. They sat quietly in the calm mental state which we call meditation and gently, but persistently, focused their attention on the concept of the temperature they wished their body to feel. This is similar to the processes now being increasingly used in the mental approach to cancer.

It is sometimes objected that many people who attempt to control or eliminate their cancer by such means do not succeed. 'There,' say the sceptics, 'I told you there was nothing in it.' But a high proportion of people who are given the most advanced orthodox medical treatment also die. We do not immediately say that such treatment is wholly wrong — only that it is not yet perfected. As research continues so each field learns more. The absurd thing is that millions are spent on research into the orthodox field, while only a handful of devoted people examine and work in the most exciting, most rewarding and wholly natural area — how we control our own body.

It is important to remember that the process is, in essence, simple. An Indian yogi, Swami Rama, now head of an institute which conducts wide-ranging research, demonstrated under laboratory conditions his ability to control his own heartbeat to an amazing degree — a process which has great implications in the natural approach to hypertension and allied problems. The approach he used was simply to sit quietly and meditate upon a blue sky, with tiny clouds which hardly moved. Fixing his concentration on this almost-still scene, he slowed down the body correspondingly with a remarkable change in the beat of the heart.

If this control has been demonstrated time and time again, why do we take so little notice? The answer was probably given by another distinguished yogi, who declared 'Human beings will do anything to help themselves — except work for it.' We are conditioned, brain-washed, into believing that others must do things for us, that we do not possess the capacity ourselves. It is an insidious process, because it relieves us of any responsibility for ourselves. We all feel our own problems are unique. So when we hear of others opposing, even conquering their difficulties we tend to say, 'That's different.' And we sit back and wait for the wonder treatment to become available. Someone physically disabled will tend to feel that changing skin temperature or the heartbeat is not immediately relevant. The pathology of their particular condition is quite different. But is it? In cases of environmental disease a framework which was originally working at least adequately has begun to go wrong. Why? Congenital or accidental difficulties may well present a different picture, but the body's amazing adaptability must never be overlooked and remarkable transformations can and do occur. We will consider this aspect in more detail in the next chapter.

2.

YOGA AND DISABLEMENT

This book is intended primarily for the physically disabled person. It therefore must be confined to what the reader can safely do on his or her own. This is not a major limitation for the whole basis of the approach can be undertaken personally, even if help is desirable.

It has to be understood that yoga is not an alternative to physiotherapy, or even a way of relaxing without taking pills. It is an appraisal of the realities of life and an examination of how we work successfully within these realities. That sounds a pretty big claim, but nothing less will satisfy. Sometimes yoga is described as a way of life, but even this is an artificial limitation. The yoga understanding of the universe and of man's place in it is quite remarkable and it has to be remembered that this understanding is wholly based upon intuition and experience. Early yogis did not have laboratories or scientific instruments or electronic instruments. They became quiet and cleansed their minds and then set down what came to them.

The remarkable thing is that this intuitive knowledge more and more matches up with modern scientific knowledge or, rather, we should put it the other way round and say that modern science, with its wealth of instruments and millions for research, is more and more discovering the truth of yoga.

Before we expand on this, let us start by examining the different forms of physical disability. Of course, disability must first of all be removed from the stigma of illness. Many disabled people are extraordinarily well. If illness is equated with something going wrong with our basic functioning, then we are all ill. There is no one whose body is not locked in combat with some potentially dangerous alien influences. This is why we have such a hard-working immune system. Everyone of us has cancer, in the sense that we all have some cancerous cells which are being killed. The illness comes only when the enemy begins to gain a foothold. So the human body is very much like the world in microcosm. The wars, revolutions and outbreaks of violence in our planet are matched by the battles constantly being fought by our bodies to repel invaders and 'rogue' cells. At a simple level we can say that environmental disability has been brought about by a pressure of dis-harmony (dis-ease) which has so upset the body's natural balance that the inbuilt health service has been unable to cope. As a result nerves, muscles or other aspects of the body's system have been affected. Some of these specific dis-harmonies are susceptible to established medical treatment and are therefore described as 'curable'. For others there is no current treatment and they become known as 'incurable'. 'Incurable', however, is a reflection upon the state of the medical profession and not a definitive statement about the dis-ease itself.

The trouble is that there is a growing realization that even the most serious of dis-eases is a symptom of something deeper and that removing the symptoms of that illness does not necessarily mean that a healthy, happy human being will thenceforth develop. This is one aspect in which the concept of yoga, concerning itself with cause, goes much deeper than the treatment of symptoms.

Others are disabled through accidents. Here a wide range of after-effects may materialize. Broadly speaking, current medical opinion holds that many of the consequences of accidents (or of strokes or heart attacks) can be ameliorated providing they are tackled swiftly and thoroughly. Appreciation is deepening of the body's immense capacity for recovery. It is, however, generally felt that such recovery is confined to the first few months after the event and then no further progress is possible.

There are enough exceptions to this rule, however, to throw serious doubt upon the validity of such limitations. After all, it is not long ago that improvements which are now taken for granted were held to be impossible. It seems likely that even accidents in which the spinal cord is severed may be seen before long as much less definitive than they are regarded as being today. An increasing number of neurologists claim that nerve cells do seek to regenerate themselves. Here again the process of self-repair is the key one, yet is sadly neglected.

Mishaps, often at birth, resulting in spasticity are now, fortunately less common; yet many people still suffer confined lives as a result of birth traumas. Cerebral palsy is certainly beyond our capacity to fight at this time; but spastics can help themselves to lead a much fuller and less stress-ridden life, if they see the natural principles involved. Fortunately, too, less children are now born with congenital deformities, although we still have the occasional scare arising from the side-effects of pharmaceuticals. Even in our wildest dreams we do not yet aspire to the generation of limbs or organs which are missing or sadly deformed, but the ability to lead a rewarding life within such disablement is much greater than we often allow.

It will be seen that expectations will vary immensely. In fact, however, the central point is not the expectations but the value of making the greatest use of that which is available; bringing greater meaning and fulfilment to life. The remarkable changes which human beings have shown that they can bring about in their body processes have occurred because the means used were wholly compatible with the end achieved; the means involved being quiet, calm and resolute. These are life qualities and go far beyond the limited objective of opposing symptoms or changing bodily functions.

Not long ago physicists regarded the universe as a conglomeration of all sorts of different systems and principles. As knowledge has grown, on the one hand the complexity has been realized to be vastly greater than ever before imagined, but on the other an equivalent simplicity has been discovered. Currently the scientist avers that everything has been reduced to three principles and the firm belief is that, given the time and the immense sums of money needed for modern research, it will not be long before these three principles are integrated into one. In other words everything radiates from a central, unifying factor, like spokes from the hub of a wheel. The implications of such a view are vast: the natural state is for everything — and everyone — to function within that single principle. The failure to follow this path promotes disharmony and dis-ease. The concept of yoga is wholly in agreement with the modern physicist's contention and it takes the implications of this unity into every aspect of life. The trouble is that in these practical, mechanized days we want only to be up and doing — and we do not really worry what it is we are doing, so long as it is something. People with a disabling disease will tend to translate this into a whole series of so-called cures, or palliatives. This way leads not to health but to greater suffering.

A single principle
A single principle indicates the need for singleness of purpose and it is significant that great teachers throughout the ages have emphasized this as the prerequisite of success. 2,500 years ago the Buddha declared:

> Set your heart in one place and nothing is impossible to you.

By using the word heart he was immediately outlawing all these modern mind-control systems which profess to offer you the ability to do anything, either good or bad. The Buddha uses the word heart as the scientist might use the phrase 'single principle' — that is, something in accord with the pattern of the universe, something which is integrative in nature and not divisive, something which is not merely seeking to enhance our own ego. 'One place' clearly determines the need for total single-pointedness. It is no good trying to achieve something when we think of it, when we feel in the mood, when we don't feel too tired, or by rushing round to try every man-devised technique which is on offer. We set our sights and we never move away from them. Finally, the Buddha declared that if the two prime conditions are obeyed nothing is impossible 'to you' — in other words, *we* achieve, we do not leave it to someone else to do it for us. This is an inspiring statement, but it should be seen as more than that: it is a statement of total scientific validity. It accords with all we know of the basic coherence of the universe.

How, then, should we face up to a problem of disablement? What should be our attitude to it? The first thing is the realization that life is much greater then the physical body. It is convenient for the body to function well. It is convenient that it should be healthy and that its working parts should move adequately. But such things are not the be all and end all of life, as many a physically disabled person has discovered.

The path and the progress of mankind are both made clear by the many amazing examples of others, which give us strength and encouragement. Prime among such examples are the achievements of countless numbers of physically disabled people. Some have so opposed their disablement as to conquer it; others have come to terms with the limitations, however severe, and have created for themselves a fulfilling lifestyle which has made them far happier and more contented than their able-bodied friends and associates. We are all aware of the more celebrated cases of each approach, but we should not think that they alone have achieved their objectives.

To give an example, a middle-aged woman living in Essex has appalling difficulties with one of her legs. Surgery failed to make the position any better and her specialist told her that she would have to wear a calliper for the rest of her life. She attended a local yoga group once a week, where she had been taught the central importance of natural breathing and she determined that she would oppose the problem by developing her energy through her breath. So she practised daily, persistently and quietly. She visualized her leg getting better as she breathed calmly and rhythmically. After a while she discovered that she no longer needed a calliper. A little later she was able to resume dancing, which had been her favourite pastime, and which she feared was gone for ever. She returned to her specialist to show him the improvement. 'Oh,' he grunted grudgingly, 'You are one of the lucky ones.' The problem leg is still thinner than the other, but apart from the need to wear boots (fashionable ones) in winter she no longer has any problem. She set her heart in one place and persisted in a natural process. Much of this book will be devoted to human energy and its development through the breath.

Others whom I know have not made any dramatic improvement in their disability because life has offered them something else instead about which to become centre-pointed and we can only work on one major objective at a time. I know several people with multiple sclerosis who have told me they regard it as the best thing that happened to them. They say this because the challenge of the problem has altered the whole direction of their lives. One woman I know has found that she can communicate with others much more deeply and her life is a full one, helping and counselling others. She gets no better — she also gets no worse. She holds her physical condition static while she gets on with the job in hand and leads a fulfilling life. How many of us with full use of limbs and organs find life fulfilling?

Controlling the mind

The more one examines every aspect of this subject, the more one realizes that one factor crops up universally — the mind. Some 2,000 years ago a great sage of yoga, named Patanjali, declared: 'Yoga is controlling the activities of the mind.' In that one sentence he summed up the whole basis of life. I have already pointed out that in our infancy the overwhelming majority of us performed the miracle of movement and co-ordination, starting to use our arms and legs and continuing to do so, with total persistence, until we mastered the process. We need to see that the life of the human being demands a second miracle — the ability to control our minds as fully as the able-bodied person can the limbs.

Of course, in these prosaic days we do not believe in traditional miracles — the instant cure — even if secretly we still long for them. Now that we know the universe is an integrated whole, processes that cut across such integration are clearly either impossible or positively harmful. The true miracle is the ability to achieve, carefully and slowly, by setting our sights on a right objective and keeping on until we have victory.

A fundamental way of looking at life is encapsulated by Richard Bach when he provides this aphorism in his book *Illusions*:

There is
no such thing as a problem
without a gift for you
in its hands

You seek problems
because you need their gifts.

Can the problem of disablement be regarded as a gift? Some disabled folk may feel anger at such a suggestion; see it as a patronizing remark from an able-bodied person. The truth is that we are all disabled, it is only the form of disablement which varies. I have often described my own disablement as creeping financial paralysis — as real as any directly physical limitation. This has been incurred by taking on the building up of an organization, with an expensive residential centre, without any grants or guaranteed income. So life is spent flirting with bankruptcy. The mental and physical consequences of such a state can be grave indeed. Yet that problem is also a gift, for it has been a constant stimulation and challenge. I have not overcome my 'illness' as yet, but I have controlled it and that provides a real sense of achievement.

I have stressed the need for quiet, calm, stillness. As with everything else in yoga this is a practical assessment, underlining a practical need. A central approach to the controlling of mental activity is the process known as meditation, which we will consider in more detail later. To many people this seems a strange and esoteric practice and one that is a little frightening. However, the process of meditation has been examined carefully and scientifically, with some surprising results.

Firstly, it has been discovered that someone meditating reduces the intake of oxygen by around twenty per cent. If, however, you come home and 'relax', by flopping into an easy chair, oxygen is reduced by no more than five per cent. Why the big difference? In each case the body is physically inactive, in fact a meditator is maintaining slightly more body tension than anyone simply relaxing. We know, however, that the biggest consumer of energy in our body is the brain, which requires some twenty per cent of our energy quotient, even though it represents only two per cent of the body's cubic capacity.

The remarkable drop in oxygen intake during meditation, therefore, is a clear indication of reduced brain activity. That brain activity is largely involved with uncontrolled thoughts and sensations passing through us like the chatter of monkeys; it is a constant drain on our energy which only produces confusion in our lives. Many a doctor has said to his patients; 'Hard work never killed anybody — it is unrelieved mental stress which does it.'

Biofeedback
In recent years an electronic process has been developed which is called biofeedback. Various ways are devised of monitoring the body's response to certain conditions. One of the simplest and most frequently used of these is a machine which checks the electrical resistance on the skin. Allowing for a numbers of factors, this resistance is an indicator of our state of relaxation or tension. The higher the resistance, the greater the tension indicated. Such machines have been used in a wide range of experiments in hospitals and elsewhere. It is normally found, for example, that the skin registers a calmer, more normal state after a person has lain down and relaxed effectively for, say, fifteen minutes.

The machine is activated by placing electrodes on two fingers and then turning a dial. At the point on the dial at which the resistance begins to take effect, a ticking noise is produced. Basically, the higher the number on the dial at which this noise is heard, the more relaxed is the state of the person being examined. If you fit the electrodes on your own fingers, switch on the machine, assess the point at which the ticking sound begins — and then proceed to make yourself feel utterly miserable, the tick will turn into a high-pitched scream. You then stop your play-acting miserable thought and become mentally peaceful again, but the scream continues, slowly diminishing, for minutes afterwards. We see, therefore, that a phoney miserable thought, maintained for only a few seconds, will produce an immediate and unpleasant change.

This change persists throughout the body — the electrodes will also react if placed on the toes! The important factor, therefore, is not whether the anxiety or fear is real or imagined. Both will affect the functioning of the body almost instantly. If maintained, the whole body process will be put into a state of unrelieved stress, thereby weakening its ability to function normally.

If the body is already weakened, let us say through the process of a disabling disease, such unrelieved anxiety brings an unnatural pressure on body systems which are less able to cope. The result is described as a relapse: all too often it is a relapse of the body simply monitoring a relapse of the mind. Few people would today disagree with the contention that the control of the mind is critical to a fulfilled and healthy life, for only by such control can unrelieved stress be obviated. How do we achieve it?

Often we have little or no idea of the stress factors working on us. A while ago I was staying in the home of a yoga teacher and was talking with her husband, a pleasant man with a modest executive job. He told me what wonderful things yoga had done for his wife. 'I don't need it,' he added. 'I'm quite relaxed. I've got my garden and I take the dog out for a walk every night. I'm OK.' One week later that man was in hospital with a nervous breakdown. How, then, can we tell the truth of our own situation? And how can we come to grips with it? Fortunately the human being has evolved with a fail-safe system, something which provides a sure foundation for our lives and upon which we can build. This foundation will be described in detail in the next chapter.

3.

THE SOURCE OF ENERGY

One can live without speech,
for there are the dumb.
One can live without sight,
for there are the blind.
One can live without hearing,
for there are the deaf.
One can live without thought,
for there are the simple.
One can live without limbs,
for there are the crippled.
But one cannot live without breath.

These wise words appear in a series of ancient Eastern manuscripts, widely quoted in yoga, which are called the Upanishads. Breath is the whole basis of life; the heart itself would not beat if the breath did not begin the process. The breath is the very basis of our thought, for it provides the energy which activates the brain; the very basis of our movement, for from it comes the energy which activates the body; and the very basis of our health, for energy is the whole fuel of life.

If we are healthy, happy and peaceful, our breathing is full and natural. All forms of ill-health, all forms of mental un-ease manifest themselves in the breath. Our mental and physical difficulties cause breathing difficulties and these breathing difficulties exacerbate the mental and physical difficulties. It becomes a vicious circle.

The person with a disabling disease suffers from

impaired breathing, caused by neuro-muscular attempts to resist the weakness or loss of balance produced by the symptoms of the disease. The breathing is further impaired by the worry and unhappiness at the knowledge of having the illness itself — quite apart from any other areas of mental tension which may exist. The person with a congenital disease has had the breathing affected from birth, again by both the physical and the psychological factors. But the wonderful thing about the breath is that we have immense voluntary control of it.

It is highly significant that there is no other body system that functions like our respiration. It is, of course, automatic — or autonomic. We do not have to remember to breathe; the brain/body relationship keeps functioning so long as we live. Yet we also have immense voluntary control over it. Normally we breathe between fourteen and sixteen times a minute: any averagely healthy person can change this to four breaths a minute — or twenty-four — just by taking a conscious decision. As mental and physical problems become more severe, so taking control of one's breath becomes more difficult — but it is never wholly impossible. Nothing else in the body functions in this way. Vital functions, including heartbeat, blood-pressure and so on, are autonomic. Largely thanks to experiments with yoga, it has been found that such functions can be affected voluntarily. Yoga processes of relaxation will calm an excessive heart rate; likewise, trials have shown that hypertension can be opposed and even conquered. All these take time, however, even in the strongest individual. Breathing changes can be effected immediately by the healthy and relatively quickly by most other people. Severe spasticity presents a problem, as does mental handicap, but even here persistence can bring surprising results.

Life is breath...
Since breath is the fuel of life, this means we have the foundation of our body/brain functioning largely within our own control. Throughout the ages, great civilizations have paid particular attention to the breath. To quote again from the Upanishads:

Life is breath
And breath is life.

For some reason our society has come largely to overlook this central truth. True, lip service is paid to 'deep breathing', but this is at a very superficial level. The truth is truly wonderful. We know that if someone loses his temper he is enjoined, 'Calm down. Take a few deep breaths.' The worst of the temper begins to evaporate. If someone is terrified, precisely the same advice is given and the fear begins to lift. Breathing does not only control body function, it affects our mental attitude and our emotions as well.

If we are to seek to combat our difficulties, whether they be mental or physical — and, in fact, all difficulties are ultimately a combination of these two factors — we must begin with the breath. Let me offer two analogies. If you buy a brand new car and wish to show it off to your friends, you will be highly embarrassed if you sit in the driver's seat, switch on the ignition and nothing happens. You will be even more embarrassed if, when the car still fails to move, you have to admit you did not know you had to put petrol in the tank. Petrol is the basis of energy for the car just as surely as breathing is the basis of energy for the human being. Similarly, if, when driving, the car begins to judder and the engine begins to cough, you check whether anything is wrong with the fuel supply. How often do we check whether anything is wrong with our fuel supply?

In recent years there has been an increasing medical realization that many symptoms of illness, previously regarded as illnesses in their own right, can now be traced back to a disruption of natural breathing. The process which has been especially investigated is hyperventilation, or over-breathing. One specialist in this area now estimates that some seven per cent of the population of Britain is affected by this problem. The commonest sign of over-breathing comes when a person constantly breathes rapidly and shallowly, in the top of the lungs, upsetting the body's essential balance between carbon dioxide and oxygen. A wide range of symptoms can follow, which generally disappear when the breathing is returned to normal.

While this is the respiratory dysfunction which has been most widely researched, it is, in fact, only one form of malventilation. In addition to hyperventilators, there are also many hypoventilators — those who persistently under-breathe. This is a common process among those who contract disabling diseases. In due course they take to their wheelchairs and life loses virtually all sense of purpose. What with the slouched position, the physical inactivity and the mental torpor, their breathing becomes miniscule. I have often had cause to say to such people, 'You've got the body of a grown human being and the breathing of a mouse!' No wonder they degenerate.

Just before writing this chapter I went to visit a lad of twenty-seven in Northern Ireland, who has multiple sclerosis. He has some difficulty in walking, brought about by poor balance and there is an occasional slight tremor in his hands. At this moment his real symptoms are relatively light. Yet he has not been out of his house in months: all through the summer he stayed indoors, moving only between his bedroom, the living-room and the dining-room. He spends virtually the whole day sitting slouched in an armchair. He watches endless television. He is miserable and feels helpless and hopeless. And he is hardly breathing. No wonder he has 'got the skids under him'. Anyone leading his life would sink and sink at an ever-accelerating rate. Naturally, his parents urge him to 'snap out of it' — but how can he? His breathing is so poor that his brain is barely ticking over. Such an under-energized instrument cannot be expected to be capable of positive and constructive thought.

Many other people exhibit their agitation by fluctuating between bursts of energy and determination and periods of sunken depression, or gusts of anger, interposed by milder periods. Examine their breathing and one finds it is like a pump which has gone dramatically wrong, so that no even flow of energy passes through the body, rather it proceeds the whole time in fits and starts, causing these sudden transformations in mood. After all, the picture and sound of your television set would be impossible if the current passing through the mains to feed it juddered constantly between 100 volts and 250 volts.

The subtle process of energization

For many years Western medical thought compared the human being to a machine. Even now the idea persists. In one sense this cannot be denied and man has certainly devised every form of working machine in his own image — and that of other living creatures whom he has observed. The energy necessary to power man-made machines must either be combusted (as in coal) or generated (as in electricity). Man's own energy is both combusted (oxygenation) and generated (again electricity). The great difference is that a person is a living machine: every single part is alive and functioning in balance and relationship with all other parts. This makes the energization of a person a much more subtle process than the energization of a machine.

If you ask people about breathing they will probably say that its purpose is to provide us with the life-giving force of oxygen and to eliminate the poison of carbon dioxide. This is only a tiny part of the truth and, strange as it may seem, even today medical research knows relatively little of the process and subtlety of respiration. Oxygen, for example, while essential to body functioning, is a toxic substance. It can be a killer! As with everything else in our body, it needs to be absorbed and used in the right quantity, with the right balance. Carbon dioxide, whilst also toxic, is not simply an enemy to be eliminated by the body. In hyperventilation, for example, the level of carbon dioxide in the body becomes too low, with damaging results.

Little attention is paid to the fact, yet it is now known that the body is also a wholly electrical organism. Every single cell has its own force field and the systems of the body are electrically receptive. The first body system to be discovered to have an electrical charge was the nervous system; yet even today the importance of the effective maintenance of this charge in cases of neurological disease does not seem to be appreciated. Because body electricity is an immensely subtle process, we as yet know little about it. This, however, emphasizes its importance in the process of our health and inner fulfilment rather than diminishes it.

Electricity plays a role, often dominant, in body

functions: the heart is an electrical pump; every message within the brain is conducted by means of electrical impulse. But it goes far beyond this. Recent research has revealed the presence of what has become known as Life Fields, L-fields for short. One of the leading researchers in this area, Professor Harold Saxton Burr, wrote: 'Most people who have taken high-school science will remember that if iron-filings are scattered on a card held over a magnet they will arrange themselves in the pattern of the 'lines of force' of the magnet's field. And if the filings are thrown away and fresh ones scattered on the card, the new filings will assume the same pattern as the old. Something like this — though infinitely more complicated — happens in the human body. Its molecules and cells are constantly being torn apart and rebuilt with fresh material from the food we eat. But, thanks to the controlling L-field, the new molecules and cells are rebuilt as before and arrange themselves in the same pattern as the old ones.'[1]

While, as yet, I am not aware of any research directly relating the body's electrical circuitry and L-fields to respiration, the relationship in fact is directly observable. I have now spent the past seven years observing the changes which effective natural breathing will bring about in people of all sorts — from the apparently able (sometimes called the 'not yet ill') to the seriously disabled. The correlation between breathing and health and mental equilibrium is so clear that the response of the body's electrical basis to ordered, full breath is obvious. It is now possible to demonstrate this, at least in part, electronically.

Thanks to the L-fields, cells and molecules do renew themselves recognizably, for example when we meet someone after a period of some months we are actually looking at a wholly different person, physically, since the cells and molecules have been renewed throughout the body during that period. But changes do take place and we need to ask ourselves why. Generally the answer is that we are older, the ageing process has set in, or that ill-

[1]   Harold Saxton Burr, *Blueprint for Immortality: Electric Pattern of Life Discovered in Scientific Break-through* (Neville Spearman, 1972).

health has made us pale and haggard. Yet it is now being realized that the ageing process is to a great extent a myth. It is our lifestyle and our physical illnesses, all too often closely inter-linked with that lifestyle, which drag us down.

So the process is this: natural respiration — basically an autonomic process — provides the whole basis of body energy. It balances oxygen and CO_2, it ensures the effective combustion of oxygen with the food we eat to make the energy forms of proteins and other essential substances. It also controls the varied electrical impulses which are basic to the whole of our life and these monitor the functioning of all aspects of the body. Naturally, I am not saying that right respiration will of itself 'cure' illness or disability, but I do maintain that without right respiration no real cure is possible. Symptoms may disappear or be suppressed, but the real cause of the trouble will remain untouched and is likely to recur, in the same or a different form. But, it may be objected, breathing is an autonomic process, even if we can control it voluntarily; surely, therefore, we should leave it alone. The fact is that autonomic processes are not unchangeable. They are reflexes, subject to modification — and even downright transformation — by a variety of circumstances.

Already I have pointed out that disabling diseases result in unnatural muscle tensions being brought into play, to overcome balance problems and diminishing power in limbs. Someone whose legs begin to fail will tense the abdominal muscles and, all too often, the lower back muscles, in an attempt to keep on the feet. Normally these muscles are brought into play quite briefly and are then allowed to relax, but diminishing physical ability can result in a permanent state of tension, which will not only induce spasticity but also affect the functioning of the whole area around. Emotional tension adds to the problem. Any sudden shock will result in our tensing up the abdominal muscles in reaction. 'Butterflies in the stomach,' we often call it. This, too, can become permanent causing resulting problems. Anxiety, also affects the upper part of the chest. Here the tension corresponds with living creatures. When we are young, a tension around the cardiac plexus will activate the heart muscles and we feel our heart pounding at the sight of a desirable member of the opposite sex. If we are going to have a difficult talk with anyone, we will find the construction in the same area. Hence the popular saying, 'My heart was in my mouth.' All these tensions, physical and emotional, damage the normal functioning of the trunk and, as a result, distort the natural autonomic breathing reflex. Thus the whole body/brain function goes 'out of sync'.

This is where the wonder of the voluntary control of the breath comes in. We have an inbuilt system of regulation which puts us firmly back in the driving seat. We have a basic control over body and mind, we are not out of control. This realization is central to the whole concept of health. Of course, restoring the natural breath is not the whole story, but it is the first essential without which we are lost. To give a metaphor here, if you look at any town or village you will see an immense variety of houses: big, small; cottage, mansion; old, new; stockbroker Tudor, block of flats. If, however, you demolish all these varied structures and see what is left you will find something of virtual uniformity: the foundations. The house may exemplify the character of its owner — but the foundations are the sure basis on which the house is built. Without them the structure falls down. So it is with our own lives, the foundation of which is the life breath.

4.

RESTORING THE ENERGY

What, then, is the natural process of breathing? To answer this question we have first of all to examine the balance of life itself.

The two basic elements of life are will-power and tension on the one hand, letting-go and relaxation on the other. Without the drive to live, life could not sustain itself. We are, in fact, told that every cell has a 'will' to live. The maintenance and continuation of life are basic instincts within us. These combine with the necessary tension to push forward, both physically and mentally. While these aspects are essential, they must be counter-balanced for effective living. If we keep up will-power, determination, tension, without relief, we shall collapse. Muscles held in tension become spastic, as many a disabled person finds when limbs go into spasm. Mental spasm is just as real a phenomenon. The ability to let go and relax is therefore equally important. Unfortunately, this is an area of life which we have lost to a great degree.

The reason for the loss is this only partly-developed aspect of mankind: consciousness. Consciousness is a wonderful thing if our minds are under adequate control. It gives us intuitive knowledge, it enables us to discriminate and decide upon our course of action. When it is not under control the result is that we 'chew over the fat', we are unable to make up our mind, we fret and worry. If an animal has a fight, once it is over it is very likely to curl up and go to sleep. In similar circumstances the human being will tend to continue to seethe; 'This is what I should have done … this is what I should have said … this is what I'll do next time.' This is a state of frustrated and resentful tension because we have a form of awareness which does not appear to be shared by animals — at least to anything like the same degree.

In the natural state, breathing builds the right will-power and tension and counter-balances it with effective relaxation. Every in-breath is a tension, because we have to draw the air into the lungs. It is therefore a symbol of continuing life. Every out-breath is a relaxation, gently allowing the air to flow out of the nostrils. The tense person cannot take an effective out-breath because mental agitation defeats the relaxed state which accompanies it.

In addition to every breath providing an active symbol of the balance between tension and relaxation, we actually breathe in different ways according to the requirement of body and brain. If we are relaxing — truly relaxing — there is no movement in the chest and the visible sign of breathing is a small movement of the abdomen — out on the in-breath and moving back on the out-breath. To activate the chest involves tensing muscles, expanding the rib-cage. This cannot be relaxation. Therefore, in relaxation, the relatively small expansion of the lungs is made possible by an equally small movement of the diaphragm — separating the abdominal area from the chest — brought about by the action of the phrenic nerves. As the diaphragm moves down, the abdomen, being relaxed, moves outwards in compensation and when the diaphragm moves up again on the out-breath, the abdomen resumes its former position. Because of physical and psychological tensions, many disabled people continue to activate the chest muscles when they are trying to relax; often, too, they maintain tension in the abdomen. The result is that no relaxation can really take place and the continuing state of tension becomes more and more damaging. It will be obvious that the state of relaxation is intended to restore the natural balance. It is therefore of immense importance.

Because little body energy and brain energy should be required in periods of relaxation, the breathing should become equally relaxed, slow and rhythmical. Body systems are 'ticking over', muscular tension is minimal. Likewise the brain is not puzzling over any major problem and even stray thoughts should diminish appreciably. Sadly enough, this seldom happens with many people. Experiments have shown that tension is maintained and the brain continues its wasteful and worrying agitation, thus countering any benefits which might come from the less active state. The 'I always feel tired' syndrome is endemic in our society.

The problem is made even worse by the fact that the natural form of energizing, breathing, has also largely been lost. When we are active, mentally and physically, our breath takes on quite a different form. Now we need energy to flow through body and brain, without either being blocked or draining away. How this is achieved can be seen by a look at the anatomy of the human trunk.

Unlike the trunk of almost all other creatures, that of the human being is designed to be held upright. The spine has two natural counter-balancing curves, the muscles are designed to support the right posture and the positioning of muscles, ribs and diaphragm are beautifully arranged for the purpose of energization. The diaphragm is the piston of the body, an extremely strong sheet of muscle, separating the lungs and rib-cage from the abdomen and visceral area. It is designed to move with the breath, not merely to allow for the enlargement of the lungs on the in-breath, but also to provide a massage and release effect on the visceral organs and to stimulate body energy by its pumping motion. Even the functioning of the heart is enhanced when the breath is natural and rhythmical. The full effect is only possible when the trunk is held erect — something which we all too seldom do these days and which becomes more difficult, though usually not impossible, in cases of disablement.

The diaphragm is attached to the bottom, or floating, ribs in the front and to the spinal column at the back. If these ribs are activated they move up and out with the result that the diaphragm is stretched, its central cone largely levels out, the lungs can expand and the abdominal area is pressed. When the breath is released, the cone of the diaphragm is resumed, the ribs coming down to achieve this, and the abdomen becomes relaxed. Or, at least that is what *should* happen.

If the trunk is not erect, the inter-costal muscles cannot fulfil their task of moving the ribs and diaphragmatic movement is therefore impaired. The greater the slouching position, the less movement the diaphragm can achieve and the lower the energy level sinks. A similar problem occurs with those who thrust out their chests, for the positioning of the ribs now results in the diaphragm being permanently stretched and again little movement is possible. Effective health, mental and physical, depends upon the ability to breathe naturally in an energizing manner and then, when necessity demands it, to breathe in a relaxed way. Many people can do neither and their lives are then largely led in limbo. As a result, effective opposition to any illness or disability proves impossible and deterioration has to set in. That may sound to be a dogmatic statement, but it is true and identifiable.

As I said in the previous chapter, the joy is that we do have a great measure of voluntary control over our breathing, with resulting control over our life and basic health. It is important, therefore, to be precise about these aspects of breathing, so we can learn to restore our own powers.

The breath of relaxation
In yoga practice, the basic breaths are often developed lying on one's back on the floor. This has a number of advantages. The back is relaxed and in the best possible position, the trunk is slightly stretched and the movement becomes easier to identify. Where lying on the floor is impractical or very uncomfortable, it is quite possible to carry out the practice sitting.

The aim is to restore a natural process which would, therefore, be carried out lying, sitting or standing, in everyday life. For the purpose of practice, non-restrictive clothing should be worn. Tightness around the abdomen or the chest should be avoided. Even tight shoes or wrist-watch straps are not sensible. Those able to lie on the floor, or to be helped on to the floor, should lie on a suitable mat

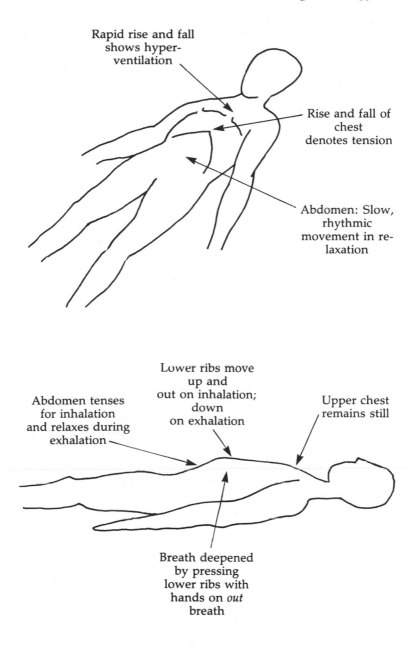

Rapid rise and fall
shows hyper-
ventilation

Rise and fall of
chest
denotes tension

Abdomen: Slow,
rhythmic
movement in re-
laxation

Lower ribs move
up and
out on inhalation;
down
on exhalation

Abdomen tenses
for inhalation
and relaxes during
exhalation

Upper chest
remains still

Breath deepened
by pressing
lower ribs with
hands on *out*
breath

Figure 1. The essentials of breathing

or rug and the area should be warm and free from draughts. Where possible, the legs should be a little apart with the ankles loose so that the toes fall outwards. The arms should be away from the side, with the palms naturally upwards. The back should be firmly in contact with the floor and the head comfortable and not to one side or the other. This, of course, is a counsel of perfection and often the best has to be made of existing capacity. However, little aids can be considered, such as putting a firm cushion between the knees to help keep the legs apart. A pillow may be placed under the back of the head where necessary, but shoulders should be encouraged to relax against the floor.

For those sitting up, the back should be as erect as possible, often a cushion in the small of the back will help there. The hands should lie gently on the lap, the head be held erect. In both cases it is best to practise with the eyes closed, as this aids peace and concentration.

To restore a relaxed breath can often be a slow process, but it is a vital and most rewarding one. If the breath is truly relaxed, the body will increasingly feel at ease and as the body feels at ease so the mind will feel more peaceful. The benefits are incalculable. To start, let us consider the ideal relaxed breath and then we can work towards attaining it. It will be rhythmical and not accompanied by tremors. The only movement will be the gentle rise and fall of the abdomen. The out-breath will be slower than the in-breath because the process of breathing out is itself a relaxation, a normalization of the body. While the breath is not deep, it will be free and unencumbered. The normal speed of fourteen to sixteen breaths a minute will be considerably reduced, to somewhere between six and nine per minute.

Remember that to try to relax is a contradiction in terms. Relaxation is the antithesis of trying. Very tense people often say to me, 'I try so hard to relax.' And when I urge them to stop trying they then declare, 'I do try to stop trying!' Moreover, relaxation is not the same as sleep. Sleep has an element of rest but it also has a number of other purposes, some of which are often anything but relaxing. In sleep, as unconsciousness takes over, we tend to breathe shallowly, largely in the top, or clavicular, area of the lungs. The abdominal movement in relaxation allows the air to permeate the whole of the lungs, with the result that consciousness is heightened, not lost. To fall asleep during relaxation is to indicate that one has not gained the art of relaxing. While I have emphasized that trying and relaxing are contradictary, in the first stages it is often necessary to pay precise attention in order to achieve the necessary groundwork.

Firstly, whether lying or sitting, one needs to be conscious of the abdominal movement. There is no question of pushing out the stomach. The movement must be gentle and natural. It is equally important to be sure that the chest is not moving. Often people are unconscious of this even when the movement is quite pronounced. It is not possible to change this actively but the mind can be brought on to the chest to help effect the stillness. With regard to the slower breathing, this can be practised when one is not actually relaxing by taking a watch and timing the breath — say between eight and ten seconds for breathing in and out again — until one becomes fully aware of this rhythm. Many people will be surprised at how much slower this is than the breath they are accustomed to take. All these preliminaries are helpful in getting the feel of relaxed breathing.

The actual practice should be for a minimum of five minutes at a time, preferably at least ten minutes. Become conscious of the gentle movement, listen to the slow rhythm of the breath and especially go with the out-breath, being aware of the sense of relaxation stealing over the body. Inevitably you will notice that this feeling is closely followed by a better state of mental peacefulness. For all of us such periods are important every day as an antidote to stress and tension.

The breath of energization

Practising the breath of energization is carried out in the same way as relaxation and most of the preliminaries will apply, especially keeping the spine erect. The importance of this cannot be over-stressed. The breath itself, however, is very different, for now muscles are activated in the chest, the intercostals, stimulating the movement of the bottom ribs. It is sensible, before beginning, to take the hands and feel where the ribs form an inverted V. This is the area which should move, not the upper chest and not the abdomen.

In relaxation the breath becomes autonomic and we consciously observe the breathing rather than consciously breathing. To stimulate energy, however, the breath is consciously developed, even though in normal life it will happen automatically. We are seeking to correct the breathing reflex and restore the natural movement which has been lost. When breathing in now, therefore, there should be a positive upwards and outwards movement of the lower ribs, but the abdomen does not inflate and the upper chest hardly moves. In this way the diaphragm moves deeply and effectively.

Many people have largely or even wholly lost the capacity to breathe in this way and they suffer accordingly. For this reason the stimulation needs to be quite strong and this can be assisted manually. The hands should be placed flat on the sides of the ribcage — *not* on top — and when breathing out they can then be pressed quite firmly towards the middle. This must be done *only* on the out-breath. Obviously this would not be done by someone who had recently cracked a rib, but otherwise it is perfectly safe provided it is confined to the exhalation. By pressing the ribs towards the middle of the trunk in this way, the breath is both deepened and lengthened. When breathing in again the hands should either be removed altogether or allowed to lie quite lightly. This stimulates the deeper in-breath and also begins to get the intercostal muscles moving again as the ribs spring out to accommodate the expansion of the lungs. This firm pressure and release with the hands will deepen and lengthen the outbreath and help restore inadequately working muscles. After a while the normal breath will improve as a result of this training.

It is extremely important not to strain after the breath. Breathing is a natural function and should be enjoyable; strain is counter-productive and must be avoided. However much one works with the breath this is an important lesson, for over-concern can create just as many problems as under-concern. Right awareness, however, helps one to adjust one's breathing at any time of stress. For example, when one wakes up out of a dream the heart is always pounding and the out-breath is more like a pant. It is perfectly possible slowly to bring this out-breath under control, by gently but firmly lengthening it. It is not easy at first because the fast panting has taken over, but conscious persistence wins the day and as the out-breath lengthens, so the agitation begins to fade away.

The same process follows everyday incidents which cause forms of stress with a resulting effect upon the respiration. If we practise and gain gentle control over these two basic forms of breathing, we have created the right foundation for our lives. Naturally, it does not mean that physical difficulties and mental worries will immediately disappear — it is not a miracle cure — but upon the breathing platform we have built for ourselves, we can now build up a more comprehensive physical and mental approach to life; this will play a major part, probably the decisive one, in combating our problems.

5.

OTHER FORMS OF BREATHING

Apart from restoring the natural breath — an essential basis for life — there are many other forms of breathing which can be helpful. The important thing is to acquire the foundation first and then build up, slowly and carefully. Do not try to do too much too quickly.

There is an excellent way of stimulating the body through breathing and demonstrating quite simply some of the many changes which effective breathing can bring about. It is a process called the Diaphragmatic Release and its aim is to achieve a deep, uninhibited breath which ensures the greatest possible movement of the diaphragm. Most effectively it is performed sitting on one's heels on the floor, but much can also be achieved sitting in a chair or wheelchair.

The person who can sit on the floor, on the heels, begins by bending deeply forward with the forearms resting on the ground, the head, quite loose, dangling nearly on the floor (*see Figure 2*). Breathe out deeply and then, breathing in, swing up, sweeping the arms up in the air above the head, coming into an upright position (*see Figure 3*). Immediately collapse down again, breathing out strongly, until once more the forearms are against the ground and the head dangling. This should be repeated, say, a dozen times. In and out breaths are both full and without any inhibition. As one comes down, the movement is not graceful but a collapse.

Someone in a chair or wheelchair can do the same thing,

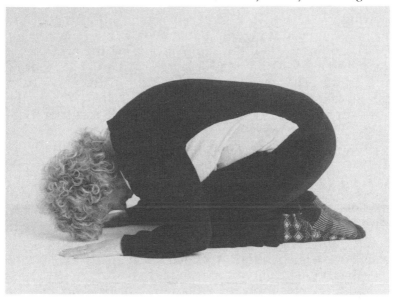

Figure 2. Diaphragmatic release breath 1

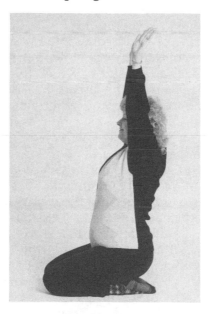

Figure 3. Diaphragmatic release breath 2

starting by resting the forearms against the thighs and leaving the head dangling just above the knees (*see Figure 4*). The action is then the same, sweeping the arms up in the air on a strong in-breath (*see Figure 5*) and letting arms and trunk collapse down on the out-breath. Obviously, care is taken to maintain balance in the chair. Where the arms do not work well, or the balance is poor, a friend can help with the movement.

Among the many changes this brings about is an increase in active muscle tone. Bring one arm out to the side at a right angle, palm down, get a friend to place one hand on the opposite shoulder, the other on the wrist of the extended arm and then get him to push down the arm while you resist as hard as you can. If this is done both before and after, a substantial increase in muscular resistance will be found. A similar strength will have come into the legs. The important thing is to realize this has been brought about simply by breathing deeply: no pill, no injection, no treatment. Of course, the enhanced muscle tone does not last for long but it is a clear indicator of how breathing does transform the body function and brain function will be similarly enhanced.

At one gathering of disabled people I was asked for help by a girl in a wheelchair who told me she had a rare neurological illness as a result of which the muscles in her arm had 'gone'. She tried this breath out in her wheelchair for the first time in her life and when she had finished I could hardly move her arm, so strong was the muscle tone. All too often we are told things with an air of authority and come to believe they are true.

This breath and some similar ones are also valuable for two other reasons: one is the removal of stale air from the lungs and the second is getting the heart pumping faster. Both are by-products of a sedentary existence, all too often overlooked. Shallow breathing, made worse by very little physical activity, often results in only the air in the top of the lungs being changed. The lower lobes tend to retain largely stale air. This not only limits breathing but also reduces the capacity of the lungs to work. One of the real dangers for the disabled person is disuse atrophy: anything in the body which is not used will begin to fail

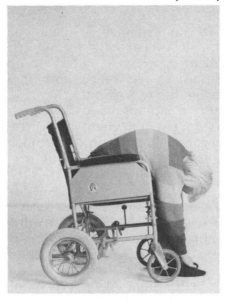

Figure 4. Diaphragmatic release breath in chair 1

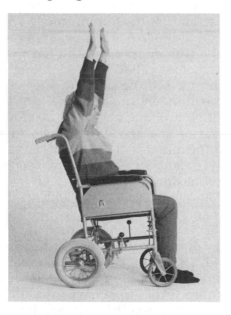

Figure 5. Diaphragmatic release breath in chair 2

and the results can be disastrous — often more serious than the original problem itself. While it would be unwise to heighten the heartbeat of someone capable of only limited movement or none at all, to too great a degree, some stimulation is desirable and these breathing processes combine the two things.

Normally the Diaphragmatic Release breath, just described, should be performed using the nostrils, for these are the proper channels for breathing. However, in clearing the lungs of stale air the mouth is opened for the out-breath and as one flops down a great, sighing 'Ha' sound is released. At the same time the abdominal muscles are contracted as firmly as possible, to push the diaphragm higher. Half a dozen of these breaths will both clear the lungs and stimulate the heart.

'Mountain' stretches
There is much talk about Deep Breathing. This is not something which is normally required, since all our physical and mental activities can usually be contained within an average breath. The value of deep breathing is to keep all the mechanism functioning and to ensure it is fully available when required. A deep breathing activity which can easily be performed either sitting on the floor or in a chair or wheelchair is called the Mountain. Sitting erect, the arms are dropped by the side and one breathes out first of all. Then, breathing in, the arms are stretched out to the sides, rising into the air and above the head, if possible just behind the line of the shoulder blades to enhance the stretch and lift the muscles of the trunk. The arms continue up until they are right above the head, touching the ears. At the point of maximum stretch it is advisable to link the thumbs, so that one is stretching right up. The lungs are now full of air and the trunk firmly controlled. After a few seconds the arms are slowly brought down again, still stretching, as one breathes out. The aim is for the movement and the breath to coincide exactly, beginning with the start of the movement and ending as the movement ends. Half a dozen Mountain stretches, performed slowly and quietly, will help lung capacity and strengthen chest and arms.

Many people with disablement, of course, will not be able to manage it fully, but regular practice, carried out thoroughly but without strain, can often work wonders. Great help in controlling breathing is provided by what is known as the Frictional Breath. This consists of breathing quite deeply as in the natural energizing breath, expanding the lower ribs, with the mouth shut. At the same time the glottis is partially closed and acts as a valve, filtering the air into the lungs. This partial closure creates a sound in the back of the throat, rather like a heavy hissing. The same process is continued with the slow, controlled out-breath. It takes a little time to achieve the sound effortlessly, but the ability to control the breath slowly and carefully is valuable.

Alternate nostril breath
It is worth describing one further breathing technique, which is called the Alternate Nostril Breath. For many hundreds of years, the yogi has realized that for much of the time we breathe mainly only through one nostril. Western medicine has only recently caught up with this knowledge. One set of experiments has shown that during the day we appear to spend about forty per cent of the time breathing through one nostril, forty per cent through the other and twenty per cent equally through both nostrils. Why? It would seem to be a part of homoeostasis — the natural energy balance within the body and it begins to give us a clue as to the fuller and deeper role which breathing plays.

The Alternate Nostril Breath evens out the whole breathing process, stimulates the nervous system and creates a feeling of calmness within the person. It has proved invaluable to many people in opposing migraine and nervous tension. The right hand is used, the right thumb being pressed against the right nostril to close it. The first and second fingers are bent down against the palm and the third finger is then used for the left nostril. Having breathed out, the thumb closes the right nostril and the breath is drawn quite swiftly in through the left nostril. The third finger then closes that nostril, so both are now closed and the breath is retained. Then the thumb moves away from the right nostril and the exhalation is carried out quite slowly through that nostril, with the left one still closed. Immediately one breathes swiftly in again through the right nostril. Both nostrils are closed and the breath retained and then the finger is removed and the slow exhalation is now out through the left nostril. This comprises one round.

The next round is begun by again breathing in through the left nostril, and so on. It is important to get the mechanics right first, so one can carry the session through calmly and quietly. Practice can initially be done therefore simply to get the finger movements correct, the breathing being added. Counting can be confusing, but the general principle is to breathe in quite speedily, retain the breath for about four times the time spent on the inhalation and then to breathe out more slowly than breathing in.

Once mastered, the Alternate Nostril Breath becomes quite easy, so the important thing is to practise slowly and get the elements together first. There is no definitive guide to the number of rounds to be taken — if at peace, your own intuition will guide you. Initially, at least, one can say not less than three and not more than ten. All the breathing methods described in this chapter are extremely helpful and there are many more available. It is most important, however, to realize that yoga is a process of calmness and control and it is useless for us to confuse ourselves with a number of different techniques. We must proceed carefully and slowly and if we do no more than restore the natural basis of breathing we have achieved the most important step. Jacks-of-all-trades are useless in yoga.

Continue, therefore, working slowly and steadily towards a natural, enjoyable breath, either relaxing or energizing as the need may be. This can be well combined with the Diaphragmatic Release breath described at the beginning of this chapter, for this helps us to breathe deeply and without inhibition and stimulates both body and mind. Whatever our difficulties, if we are alive we have to breathe. So it is only a simple step to progress from breathing to live and breathing to stimulate life and health.

6.

THE MECHANICS OF MOVING

We are now ready to consider the whole process of movement: how we move; why we move and the relationship of our movement with the breath and the mind. The impatient person may well urge: 'Well, get on with it. Cut the cackle and get to the action.' Impatience, however, is tied up with the restless mind and the process of yoga is opposing that restlessness, so we must work more slowly and in due order. To pander to the impatient is to condone the unquiet mind and that way lies disaster.

I have spoken of the miracle we performed when we were babies, in changing from uncoordinated bundles into youngsters who could use and co-ordinate arms and legs. We did it without lessons and basically without help; we did not work it all out for ourselves and apply logic or reasoning to the process. Virtually everyone knows the story of the centipede who was asked which leg it put first and became so confused that it fell over. This is an important moral tale to us, because human beings begin to lose control of their limbs when they move from autonomic movement to worried conscious movement. The able-bodied man, asked to walk very slowly and to think precisely about every movement he takes, is quite likely to fall over.

Even the autonomic process of movement is a combination of brain, breath and body — the important three Bs. The brain instructs the autonomic system to function and these instructions include information for the respiratory area of the brain on the form of breathing required. For example, if we are suddenly presented with a mental problem an urgent message is sent, changing the breathing pattern, to establish the right flow of energy to the neurones to achieve the necessary degree of concentration. Voluntary control, the use of our consciousness, is the most wonderful asset of mankind, if it is understood and applied correctly. If not, it becomes a tyrant making life more and more difficult for us.

Let us consider this in a little more detail. Those who have normal use of the arms can try an experiment. Sit at a table and place one forearm and hand quite limply on the table. Become aware of your breathing and feel it is rhythmical and quite deep. Then know you are going to raise the arm, but do not specify when. Let it rise up when the autonomic functioning of the brain tells it to. Repeat this two or three times. Now pay attention to your breathing and let it happen again. The odds are that you will find you have raised the arm while breathing in and not while breathing out. This is because arm-raising creates a modest tension in the muscles, while breathing out relaxes them. If now you experiment deliberately in raising the arm, first as you breathe in and then as you breathe out, you will find the arm feels heavier if you raise it when breathing out. By limiting the consciousness of the action and making it as automatic as possible, you will also realize that the act of raising the arm involves very little muscle tension. Mostly what is needed is good tone in the muscles, not the ability to create tension. The two main aspects of muscle activity are tonal, which is the ability to maintain muscles steadily in the minimal state of tension required for the activity, and phasic, the ability to incept the action.

Keeping the forearm lying on the table, now tell yourself the muscles in that arm are badly affected and it is very difficult, if not impossible, to raise the arm. Then try to raise it. If you put an effective message of 'I can't do it' into the brain, either you will just give up or you will put an immense effort into raising the arm. You will tense all the muscles down that side of the neck, the shoulders, the upper arm, the forearm, the wrist, the palm and the fingers. The effort will be so great that you can hardly make any movement at all. You will have made yourself — temporarily — a disabled person by the power of the mind. Exactly the same process can be carried out with the legs, or indeed any part of the body. Worry yourself about your speech and speech soon becomes impossible. Worry yourself about your eyes and they move out of focus. Worry yourself about your hearing and it becomes blurred.

The process of maintaining, restoring or enhancing our natural body movement, therefore, involves making the greatest possible use of the autonomic process, where necessary assisting this by quiet, conscious encouragement. Here is a good example of my contention. A short while ago I visited a man with severe multiple sclerosis, taking the form of intense intention tremor. Sitting in a chair, if he tries to use his arms they flail about without control. I brought with me a card of greeting from some of his friends and I gave this to him. The card was in a quite tight-fitting envelope. The tremor was so bad I had to take his hand and place the card in it to enable him to hold it at all. While he had the card, in its envelope, in his hand, I and two others in the room started to chat with him about other matters. While we did so he took the card out of the envelope all by himself! This is why ataxia is called intention tremor — it is a conscious disruption of an autonomic process. Of course, there is damage to the nervous system causing it in the first place, but the body's capacity to oppose and possibly even overcome that damage is seen when the conscious anxiety is removed and the autonomic process takes over.

Tension caused by anxiety
Neuro-muscular tension, caused by anxiety, plays a damaging role in the lives of us all. The moment we are asked to perform a physical action with which we are not familiar we begin to tense up, making the performance of the action more difficult. This can be seen in countless yoga classes for able-bodied people, where immense psycho-physical stress can be seen in people trying to do a movement of which they are a little scared. This I designate as 'yoga for stress' — or how to make yourself ill

by the practice of yoga! The fact is that we can twist anything if we want to. This is why it is so important to understand the right process from the start.

In disablement the problem is magnified. Those with congenital problems, or definitive disablements, such as paralysis, will be less liable to strain for movement they know they cannot achieve. Often they will be ingenious in devising alternative movements and making them a part of their autonomic pattern. The difficulty is very real, however, for those with disabling diseases who can never be quite sure how severe the actual damage is, who will be hoping for improvement and be all too likely to strain unnecessarily, and often damagingly, to secure movement.

Yoga is extremely important here, for the whole concept of yoga is based upon conservation of energy. When we work physically in yoga we aim at securing the best result with the least possible tension. This is one of the aspects which makes the yoga concept of movement so important for physically disabled people. The process must be faced quietly and calmly and not rushed into. Those who have great difficulty with legs and arms should be content to spend a great deal of time simply visualizing movement in affected limbs.

The movement or manipulation of defective limbs by another person does play a part in rehabilitation, but it is a very small one for the only fundamental process is that between brain and body (with the breath assisting). If someone else manipulates a limb it may secure the actual movement but the brain will have switched off and the person's own chain of command is no nearer being re-established. The same thing applies when, for example, one arm appears not to work and the person with this difficulty then always moves that arm by allowing the other hand to take it and move it. This again is necessary sometimes but it cannot be really helpful for the brain now establishes the new autonomic pattern that, say, to move the right arm the left arm is brought into action and the idea of direct action with the right arm is switched off. Of course the correct path is slow and can be wearisome, but the fact remains that it *is* the correct path and generally the disabled person has plenty of time to practise correctly. Whenever using the body, therefore, whether in everyday life, or for exercising, or for yoga postures (which are not actually exercises), always remember the three B's: brain, breath and body. The dictum to recall is that nothing in our lives is purely physical or purely mental: everything is an inter-action of mind, energy and the physical entity. By the correct use of breathing and mental relaxation I have seen people move legs, with control, which have not moved in years; I have seen people get up from the floor unaided for the first time in years. Once the inhibitions are removed, the body's real powers can reveal themselves and then we can begin really to examine the possibility and the areas of progress. Before, therefore, we come to actual movement let us consider this whole process of visualization.

Visualization
Earlier on I spoke of how yogis have been shown as able to control their temperature and their heartbeat through a process of visualization. From this we learn that if the mind is applied consistently and more intensely than the promptings of sensory stimulus, then it will take over the process of brain reaction and largely control it. This is a most important realization for it extends the frontiers of our control over our own lives. We do not know how widely these frontiers extend, but trying to find out is the greatest of challenges and truly exciting. For the present I am concerned with visualization as a process of aiding body function and movement, for by understanding and practising this we can then obtain the greatest benefit from specific movements and exercises.

To begin, therefore, we will remain sitting. Even here, however, there are always necessary pre-conditions, the most important of which is sitting erect. For many this will now be extremely difficult, temporarily even impossible, especially when it is emphasized that the sitting up needs to be relaxed and balanced and not stiff and tense. Whether sitting in a chair or a wheelchair, first of all try to ensure that the chair itself has an upright back and, wherever possible, fit a small cushion in the small of the back for comfort and balance. Then try to lift the muscles of the upper trunk and the shoulders (not shrugging, but lifting them) so the whole of the trunk is extended a little. This should be done several times so the squashed feeling, especially in the abdominal area, is reduced. So much vital activity goes on in the region of the abdomen that this alleviation of pressure is most important. Next, try to rotate the shoulders, several times to the front and several times to the back. This is to ease stiffness in the shoulderblades.

Now undertake some gentle movements of the head. Breathe in and, as you breathe out, slowly turn the head to the right. Stop when the out-breath stops. Breathe in again and when you next breathe out turn a little further to the right. Stay in this position and take several more slow breaths, allowing the neck and shoulder muscles to relax as you breathe out. Then breathe in again, turning the head to the front and, as you breathe out, turn the head to the left. Repeat the same pattern, firstly turning the head on the out-breath and then relaxing the muscles on the out-breath. Having breathed in and brought the head back so you are looking to the front, now drop the chin on the chest as you breathe out.

For the next few breaths you allow the head to drop forward on the out-breath, stretching the muscles at the back of the neck. As you breathe in, bring up the head and let it drop back. Clench your jaw and now, each time you breathe out, let the head fall back a little more, stretching the front of the neck. Finally bring the head upright again. Now bring your hands together on your lap, close your eyes and, maintaining the erect posture, begin to breathe with slow relaxation. Remember the chest is to be still and the abdomen gently moving out on the in-breath and back on the out-breath. Listen to the breath and feel that it is quite uninhibited and free, also that it is rhythmical. Pay special attention to hearing the breath move slowly through the nostrils as you breathe out. Do not be in any hurry. Time does not matter.

For a first visualization I am going to suggest a general process, so that the whole idea can be understood. As I have already pointed out, breathing is the basis of creating and stimulating energy: it takes in the raw materials of potential energy and converts them into forms essential for use within body and brain. Having begun to breathe in this quiet and relaxed fashion, with the body in the best possible position, now move to being more specific about your breath. First, feel the cool touch of the air on your nostrils as you breathe in. Except on the warmest of days the air outside is cooler than body temperature and so the first change we have to bring about is warming the air to meet our internal requirements. This is why we should breathe through the nose. The nostrils are equipped with fine hairs, cilla, which filter much of the dirt and germs out of the air and the whole nasal process is designed to bring the air up to body temperature. Normally we are not aware of this cool touch on the nostrils, but when we apply our minds to it we realize that this process is actually going on all the time.

When we have thoroughly accustomed ourselves to this process, we can turn to the out-breath and feel the warm flow of air through the nostrils. Take your time; do not rush; become one with your breath. Once you have moved into this oneness you can begin to notice that as you breathe in there is a feeling of energy flooding into the head and as you breathe out this feeling flows down through the body. Now give yourself wholly to this sensation — the energy flowing up through the head on the in-breath and down through the body, right to the toes, on the out-breath. Aided by the feeling which comes, you can now visualize the sensation as a flow of energy and identify with this flow. When any other thought intrudes, calmly push it away and come back to unity with the flow of energy throughout the body. As you practise, the stray thoughts will become fewer and are more easily dismissed. You will have a greater feeling of control and unity and this, in turn, will enchance the feeling of energy.

When the time comes to move out of this experience, first of all bring your mind back to the cool touch of the air as you breathe in, the warm flow as you breathe out and then slowly allow awareness of your surroundings to return, finishing up with the best stretch you can manage. Never come too swiftly out of such a state. How long?

There are no rules but most people will find ten minutes around average to feel benefits, although they come more speedily. Twenty minutes is quite possible, probably not much longer than that is needed for effectiveness. This process is not illusory, not merely a pretty imagining. We actually induce changes for the better within our own body systems, providing we are quietly relaxed and free from any straining.

Nearly five years ago, working with a heavily-disabled person, I had the misfortune to have my zygomatic arch broken by a spasm of ataxia on the person's part. This arch is a part of the cheek-bone. X-rays revealed a clear fracture and I was offered an operation, which I refused. After a couple of days at home (on the second of which I went out and had lunch with my wife), I returned to work. That morning we were doing some electronic testing of disabled people, together with a research doctor. I still felt a little woolly from the shock and had to catch a plane for Belfast that afternoon. I therefore suggested that I should submit myself to the type of test we were using on the disabled. This consists of checking the electrical receptivity of the body's tissue fluid, which varies in consistency — and therefore also in its electrical receptivity — according to a number of factors, principally those of the person's state of health. On subjecting myself to this process it was discovered that most of my body was functioning normally, but the area around the damaged cheek-bone was way below normal. This was to be expected as the shock of the incident had upset the normal functioning of this part.

After this reading was taken, I spent five minutes breathing quite deeply, using the ribcage as earlier described, and visualizing with each breath that the energy was flowing into the cheek. A further electronic reading was taken and found that precisely this had happened. The chart which was produced was now normal, save only for an indication that the energy was being used up quickly and it was therefore important to pay much more attention to my breathing than normal. The fractured cheek cleared up in ten days and has never given any trouble. Not a major incident, but I was sixty-one at the time and many doctors would have shaken their heads at the slowing down of body processes, making the re-knitting of the bone more difficult. Bone reconstitution and repair is known to be an electrical function of the body and therefore, by the process of effective breathing, I was stimulating the body's natural process. No medication of any sort was involved, not even an aspirin! Breathing and visualization work closely together and the more we practise and understand the process, the better the results become.

Apart from the general visualization, which I have already outlined, the process can be used as a form of stimulation for specific parts of the body. The key factor is gentleness (with oneself) and single-pointedness. At first these things can be difficult, but they improve steadily. The very first benefit is a feeling of well-being, but this is not merely a placebo, it is working steadily towards creating a situation in which the mind can be used to stimulate the body's natural functioning. The body's immune system is a remarkable process of self-help and self-health, constantly working to rid the body of invaders and rogue cells and organisms. Recently it has been suggested that some disabling illnesses involve a process in which the immune system itself is affected, thereby creating rather than opposing ill-health. It is however, perhaps significant that this concept has been developed at a time when it is acknowledged that stress factors in illness play an enormous part. It is possible that these breakdowns of the immune system, if in fact they do occur as has been suggested, may be influenced, or even directly brought on, by stress factors which become intolerable. If this is so, then the process of normalization and encouragement which is involved in relaxed visualization assumes even greater importance.

7.

THE PRACTICE OF MOVING

The Oxford Dictionary defines the relevant use of the word exercise as being 'movement of muscles, joints, etc., esp. for health's sake'. Alternatively, the word indicates a form of discipline. This second definition more correctly fits the yoga movement or posture, with the health aspect as a bonus.

There is considerable evidence that yoga physical activities provide remarkable health benefits, but this stems not simply from the movements themselves but from the total way in which they are performed. Yoga as a philosophy and practice (or perhaps a philosophical science is a better description) has evolved over some thousands of years. For the bulk of this time no specific body movements were connected with it. The technical word is *asana*, which means 'holding a position'. This referred to ways of sitting on the ground in which the body could be held correctly and comfortably. The best known of these is the 'Lotus Position', which children find easy but most adults have to practise a long time before they achieve. Yoga being the process of quietening the mind, it was quickly found that such a process depended upon finding an appropriate way of holding the body while becoming quiet and centre-pointed. Chairs being the exception, it was natural to find these positions sitting on the ground. The early Egyptians, too, practised mental control and they often used straight-backed chairs for the purpose. So while the practices differ, the essential elements remain.

About one thousand years ago a new form of yoga evolved and was given the name Hatha Yoga. 'Ha' and 'Ta' are symbols in the Sanskrit language for the sun and the moon, while the word 'hatha' means force, in the sense of a polarized force. The sun and the moon, similarly, are linked with positive and negative electrical forces, so Hatha Yoga is a process of harnessing the natural force, or energy, within the body. The aim is still the one great aim of yoga — and, in fact, of man — to control the mind. Now that the psychosomatic nature of much illness is realized and the reaction of the mind is also understood to play a key role in the progress of virtually all illness, the importance of the yoga aim can be more fully appreciated. When, therefore, considering the *asanas* or postures of yoga, never forget the depth of their intent. When a yoga activity helps a leg to move again, or eases an aching back, it is all too easy to think solely of the alleviation of the symptom — of far greater importance is the fact that the cause is being tackled.

Readers of this book will vary tremendously in their initial physical ability, but one of the pleasures of yoga is that it can be adapted to suit almost every condition. As you become more involved in the principles behind the movements, so you will be able to make your own adaptations. Broadly I will try to show how many actions can be carried out both by those who can work from the floor and those confined to a wheelchair. But consider the movement, what it is intended to achieve and then modify it to your own condition.

(i) Breathing and stretching

Stretching is important to all of us; linking the breathing with the stretch is equally important; adding mental composure completes the trinity.

Lying (Figure 6):
On one's back, with the feet together and the arms by the side, palms down. Breathe out and, as one breathes in, raise the arms slowly, stretching them, until the back of the hands touch the floor behind the head. Keep stretching and pull down on the toes, so that the whole body is extended. Then, equally slowly, stretch the arms back to their original position on the out-breath.

It is important that movement and breath coincide and that it is slowly and almost meditatively performed — that means not by thinking of the movement but *feeling* it as an integrated whole.

If the arms will not come right back, do not worry but let them hang at the final point, retaining the breath for a few seconds, so their weight can help bring them down.

This movement should be repeated several times, always with complete integration.

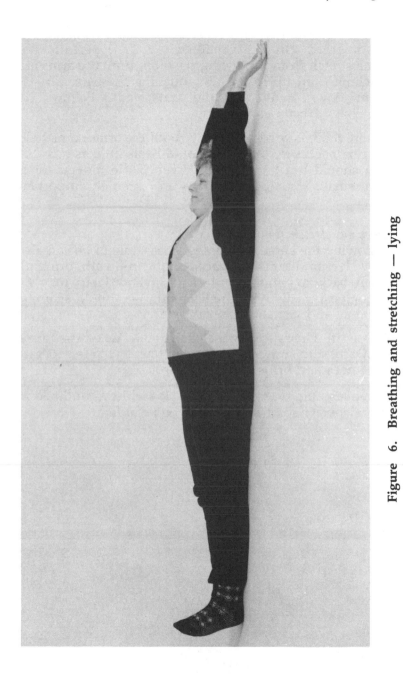

Figure 6. Breathing and stretching — lying

Sitting:
Erect, with the hands, palms down, on the thighs. On the in-breath (having breathed out first) perform the same stretch from the sitting position, until the arms are reaching right up in the air, touching the ears. Stretch them down again on the out-breath. Follow the principles exactly as for lying.

Where there is severe difficulty with the arms some help may be necessary but this should be as little as possible and should not be constant. Even if the movement is very small, visualization plays an extremely important part.

Sideways stretch (Figure 7):
Following the same principles, those able to lie can also move legs and arms outwards on the in-breath, bringing them back together on the out-breath. Help may be needed especially with the legs, but this should again be minimal and visualization maximal.

Those in chairs or wheelchairs can raise the arms outwards and stretch at the same time, trying to separate the knees and bring them outwards also.

The movements for shoulders, neck and head outlined in the previous chapter should also be included.

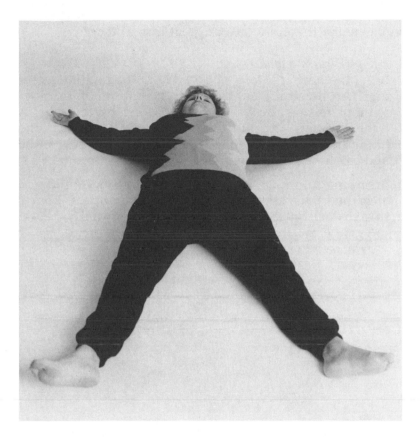

Figure 7. Breathing and stretching — sideways stretch

(ii) Working the back

The stiffening up of the back is a problem for able and disabled alike. The sedentary life of the disabled person, however, makes it more serious and often induces other problems, making life more difficult still. These movements, therefore, are of great importance.

Lying (Figures 8 and 9):
Bring the heels as close as possible to the bottom, knees together. Breathing out try to lift the bottom off the floor without raising the back. This is done by tensing the thigh muscles and the lower abdominal muscles and tilting the pelvis up. The palms are against the ground and can assist the movement.

Breathing in, bring the bottom back on the ground and arch the back, resting on bottom and shoulders. Repeat this several times enjoying the movement of the back, the gentle rocking movement soothing the mind.

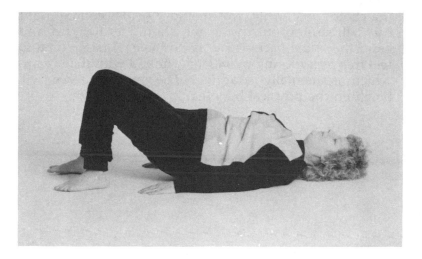

Figure 8. Working the back — lying 1

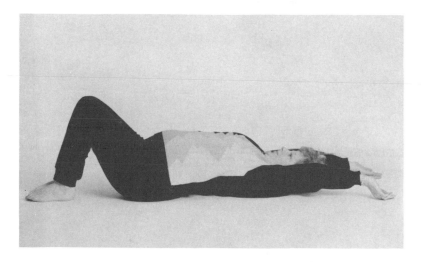

Figure 9. Working the back — lying 2

Sitting (Figures 10 and 11):
Place the hands on the arms of the chair to assist the movement. Breathing in, arch the back forward, holding the chair arms firmly, the shoulder blades coming right back. Breathing out, bring the shoulders forward and bend the spine back as far as possible. Again, come to feel this as a rocking movement, linked with the breath, which is mentally soothing. The mental peace will heighten the physical benefits.

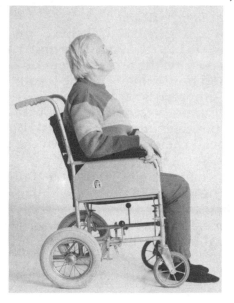

Figure 10.   Working the back — sitting 1

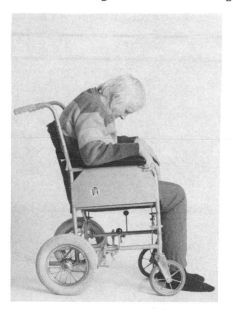

Figure 11.   Working the back — sitting 2

On all-fours (Figures 12 and 13):
Those who can get, or be helped, on all-fours can perform the slightly stronger movement known as the Cat. In this position the arms and legs do not move, only the trunk and head move with the breath. Breathing in, the back is dropped as far as possible, while the head is raised into the air; breathing out, the back is brought up as high as possible, bent in the dorsal, or middle, area, while the head comes down between the arms.

All these movements can be carried out a number of times and, indeed, need to be performed without any eye on the clock or feeling of haste. Over quite a short period of time the improvement in the state of the back will be marked and the mental benefit will also become apparent.

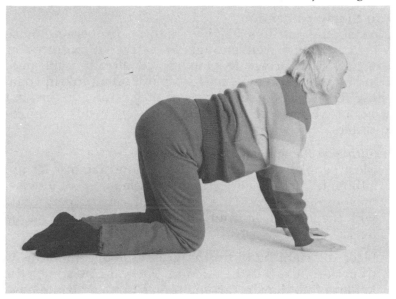

Figure 12. Working the back — on all fours (the Cat) 1

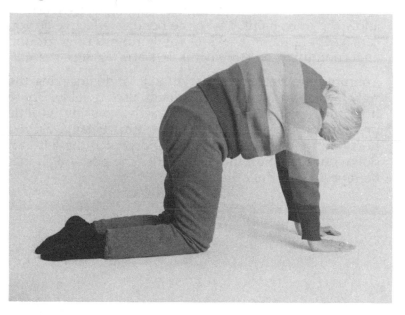

Figure 13. Working the back — on all fours (the Cat) 2

(iii) Sideways bending
No standing postures are given in this book, because those who can stand well enough to carry out postures or exercises have access to many books already published. Bending the body sideways has an important role in yoga; those who cannot stand often feel they cannot do this, but it is not wholly true. Modified sideways bends are quite possible.

Sitting on the ground (Figure 14):
Most people who can lie on the ground can also sit up, although occasionally support, human or otherwise, may be necessary. This movement can be performed with the legs out in front, cross-legged, or sitting on the heels.

Place the right hand on the ground about a foot away from the body. Breathe out and, breathing in, stretch the left arm into the air, turning the palm towards the head and continuing until the arm touches the ear. Now lift the left shoulderblade as high as possible and then, breathing out, bend to the right, bending the right arm to allow the movement. Make the bend as effective as you can, keeping both cheeks of the bottom on the ground and continuing to stretch the left arm against the ear.

You are now stretching the left side and squeezing the right, while the bend in the spine is also valuable. Try to hold this position for several breaths, putting as little pressure as possible on the right arm. Finally, as you breathe in, straighten up again and stretch the left arm down once more on the out-breath. The position should be repeated on the other side.

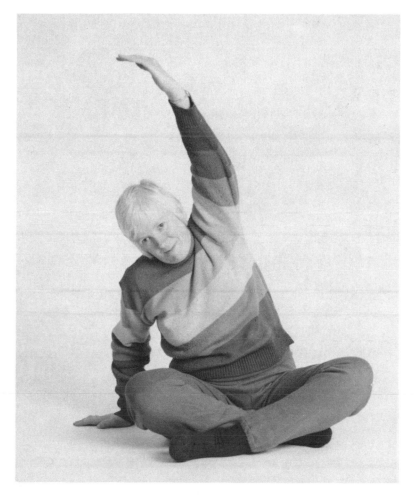

Figure 14. Sideways bending

Sitting in a chair (Figure 15):
If not in a wheelchair, it is probably best to use a chair with arms. The right forearm can then be placed on the right arm of the chair. This apart, the movement is precisely as for those sitting on the ground.

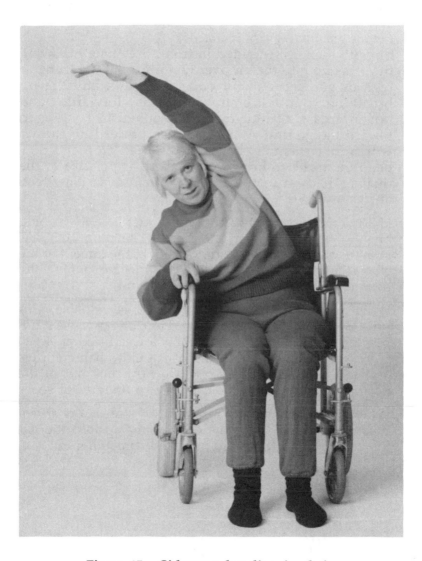

Figure 15. Sideways bending in chair

(iv) Forward bending

Once movements like the Cat and the other ways shown of making the back more flexible have been mastered, more effective forward and backward bending can be practised.

On the ground (Figures 16 and 17):
Sit with the legs extended in front. Breathing in, swing the arms up into the air over the head. Lift the trunk as high as you can and jut out your chin a little. Then, breathing out, stretch the arms forwards and downwards, stretching the back (not initially bending it) toward the ground. When you can proceed no further with a fully-extended back, let the head drop and now bend the trunk to bring you as close as possible to the thighs. Hold on to the furthest comfortable part: feet, ankles or shins.

Hold quite firmly, breathe rhythmically and as you breathe out pull with the hands, keeping the legs straight on the ground and not bent at the knee. Let the elbows move a little outwards so you are pulling the head and shoulders closer to the ground.

While the initial stretch of the back is valuable, this posture should not be maintained too long because it can put too strong a tension on the lower back muscles. However, remember that the back enjoys being supple and will welcome your work. Do not come out of the position quickly; try to hold it for two minutes or so.

When you do come up, repeat the stretch on an in-breath, swinging the arms once again up into the air. Eventually bring them to your sides, breathing out.

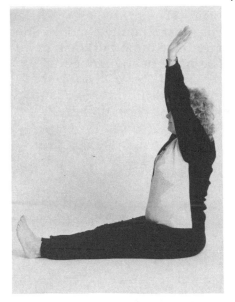

Figure 16. Forward bending 1

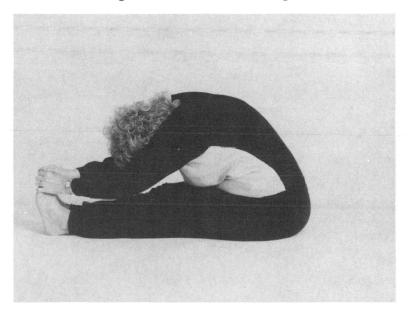

Figure 17. Forward bending 2

Sitting in a chair: (Figure 18)
Obviously this must be quite a modification. If possible, put the legs (or have them put) on a pouffe or low stool so they can be more nearly straight. Then carry out the posture as described above. Even if the legs have to be left in their usual position there is sufficient benefit to make the movement worth doing.

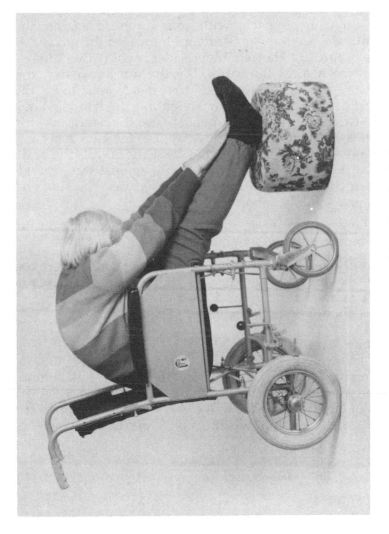

Figure 18. Forward bending in chair

(v) Backward bending

Whenever you try to stretch and bend the back forward, it is important also to bend it backwards.

Lying on the ground (Figure 19):
Lie on your stomach, with your forehead against the ground. Place the palms of your hands on the ground at the point of the shoulderblades, with the elbows pressing against the trunk. Breathe out and when you breathe in begin to raise the head and then the shoulders, without putting weight on the hands. When you can move no further, begin to use the hands, as little as possible, to help you move up. Let the back relax and do not raise the trunk higher than the navel, the body from this point down being firmly against the ground. Make sure the elbows are still tucked into the side and the arms will be bent.

If the arms are weak, the forearms may be kept on the ground at all times.

Retain the breath, holding the position, and when you breathe out come down, now doing the movements in reverse until the forehead touches the ground.
This should be repeated three or four times.

Sitting in a chair (Figure 20):
Sit as firmly as possible. Breathe out and, breathing in, bring the arms round the back of the chair to link behind. Pull against the chair arching the back and letting shoulders and head move backwards. Reverse the movement as you breathe out. Repeat three or four times.

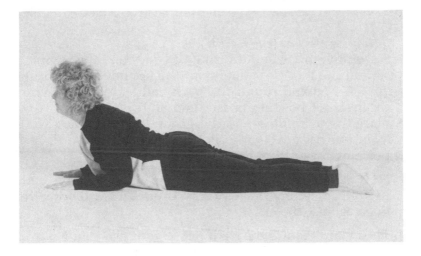

Figure 19.   Backward bending

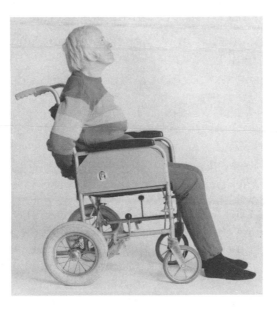

Figure 20.   Backward bending in chair

(vi) Twisting the spine

Spinal twists are extremely important physically and can save an immense amount of back trouble. The variation of pressure and release in the abdominal area is also valuable.

Sitting on the ground (Figure 21):
Sit with your legs out in front of you. Bend the right leg so that the foot is parallel with the left knee-joint. Bring your right hand round the back and feel your spine to confirm the position of the middle of your back. Now place the palm down on the ground a few inches away from the back, keeping that position, with the fingers pointing away from you.

Next take the left arm and bring the elbow over the bent right knee, letting the hand just drop. This will bring the knee against the chest.

Turn your head to the right, close your eyes, and as you next breathe out swing your shoulders firmly to the right. Try to make them parallel with the left leg. Make sure you are balanced on each cheek of the bottom. Now the lower back will feel a firm twist in that area.

Breathing quietly, hold the position for a minute or two before straightening up.

Now repeat the position on the opposite side.

Sitting in a chair (Figure 22):
If you can cross the legs, this is helpful, though not essential.

If the right leg is crossed over the left bring the right arm over the back of the chair or the top of the chair and press firmly, so that your shoulderblades swing round to the right. Close your eyes and hold the position, maintaining the best possible twist. Hold for a minute or two. Resume the normal sitting position and do the whole thing over again, using the other side of the body.

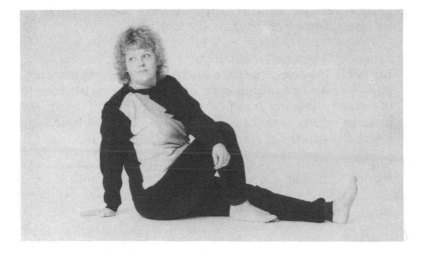

Figure 21. Twisting the spine

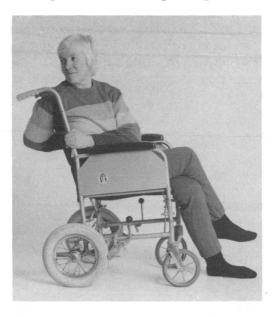

Figure 22. Twisting the spine in chair

(vii) A helpful squeeze
This movement is sometimes known as the Gas Expulsion posture. It is not an elegant title, but good abdominal pressure is important and 'wind' often plays a disproportionate part in disablement.

Lying on the ground (Figure 23):
Lie with the legs together and the hands by the side, palms down. Breathing out, bring up the right knee to the chest, link the hands around the shin, pulling the knee in tighter and then bring up the head to touch the knee. Breathing in, bring the leg back on to the ground.

On the next out-breath, bend the left knee and follow through the same procedure. Finally bend both knees. The whole process should be repeated two or three times.

Sitting in a chair:
Bring the hand together behind the right knee and, breathing out, lift the knee to the chest and bow down to try to bring the head to the knee. Breathe in as trunk and leg return. Follow the same process with the left leg. If possible, try also with both legs. Do not risk loss of balance. Repeat two or three times.

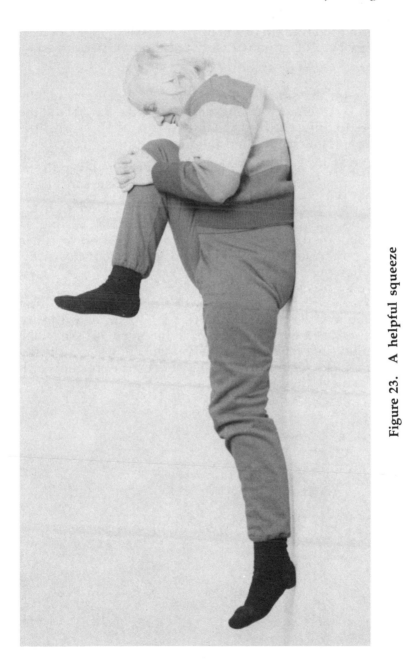

Figure 23.   A helpful squeeze

(viii) A modified Bow *(Figure 24):*
This is a modification of the Bow, a classical yoga posture. It is very helpful in many cases but cannot be performed by those in a chair.

Lying on the stomach, bring the feet together with the arms by the side, palms up. Breathing out, bend the knees to bring the heels as nearly as possible against the bottom. Now try to hold the feet.

Take a deep in-breath, then as you breathe out pull the feet strongly up, raising head and chest at the same time.

A supple person will be able to pull the thighs off the ground, as well as lifting the head and chest, resting on the abdomen. Do not concern yourself with how much you can achieve, however. Hold the position for a few seconds only. Repeat twice more.

This is one of a few yoga positions where the strong movement is done on the out-breath. Normally the in-breath is used where tension is involved or the chest expanded. In a really strong movement, however, it is the relaxation of the muscles after a deep in-breath which helps achieve the best result.

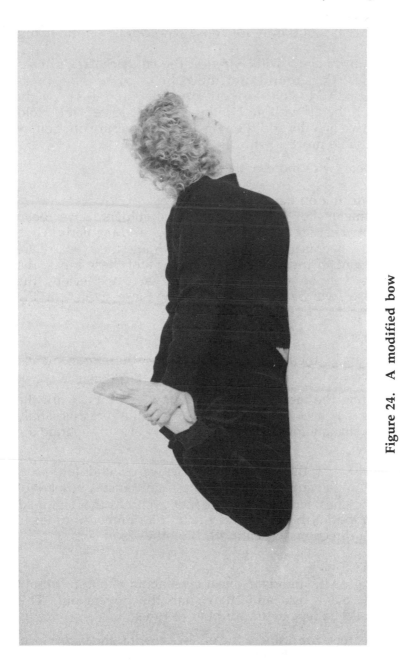

Figure 24. A modified bow

(ix) A modified Locust *(Figure 25):*
Another position only for those who can lie on the floor.

Again it begins with lying on the stomach. The chin is against the ground and the palms, by the side, press downward to give support. Breathing in, raise the right leg in the air without bending it at the knee joint. Hold for two breaths and then lower on an out-breath. Follow the same process with the right leg.

Repeat twice more with each leg.

(x) Working on hands, feet and eyes
Movements for the head and shoulders have been indicated earlier and these should be used regularly. Here are movements for the feet, the hands and the eyes. All are important. If there is difficulty in any of these areas, the effects will be beneficial. If they are unaffected, the exercises will be a way of keeping these parts working well.

Feet:
Naturally, the feet should be bare for these movements. They are best performed in a sitting position.

Placing the feet so they point upwards, first work the toes only backwards and forwards. Continue this calmly and steadily for a minute or two. Try also to separate the toes.

Next work the whole foot backwards and forwards, freeing the ankle. Ankle stiffness can cause a number of difficulties. Finally, take one foot over the other leg, hold that foot in the hand and rotate it a number of times in each direction. Repeat with the other foot.

Hands:
Bringing the hands to chest level about a foot in front of you, make fists and then snap the fingers out. This should be repeated a number of times.

Now raise the arms so the elbows are at right angles from the trunk, the hands pointing straight up into the air. Straighten the arms by snapping out the forearms.

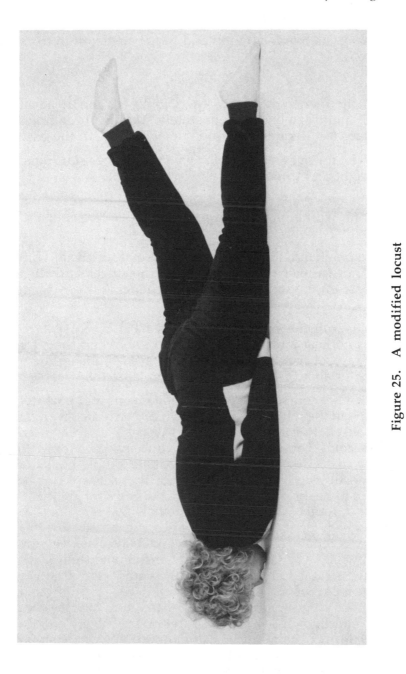

Figure 25. A modified locust

Repeat several times.

Now let the hands go limp and flap them about in front of you.

Eyes:
Look up, then to the right, down, to the left and up again — all quite slowly and deliberately. Do this three times starting to the right and three times starting to the left.

Now let the eyes slowly roll, again three times starting to the right and three times slowly to the left.

Look up to the top left and then zig-zag the eyes down and up working across to top right — and back again. Also three times.

Place one hand about a foot in front of your chest, with the index finger raised. Focus on the finger and then sharply on the wall behind. Keep changing the focus in this way.

Finally, rub the palms together as hard as possible to generate heat and an electrical current. When they are really warm clap them on the open eyes and keep them there for about two minutes. Do not close the eyes.

There are, of course, many other movements and postures in yoga but the foregoing, together with the hints given for a visualization session, can form the basis of a balanced programme. Those with greater capacity have only to acquire one of the many quite adequate simple books of yoga postures. Having worked with these it will not be difficult to adapt new ones to personal physical ability.

Never forget how these movements are to be approached. Do not see them simply as exercises, for this will be to reduce their value tremendously. Each session must therefore be tackled carefully and thoughtfully.

I have stressed earlier that yoga is understanding the development of natural balance between tension and relaxation. This should be carried through in any session. Relax, effectively, between postures. Work slowly and do not strain. Let the mind be calm and do not worry about time or external distractions. How long and how often you should practise must be a matter of personal decision.

Regularity is important. Few people cannot set aside half an hour a day for breathing and movement — separately and inter-linked. If the same time of day can be maintained, all the better. In the same way that the body grows to anticipate food at regular hours, so it will begin to expect physical and mental activities at hours it has become used to. This will always help the practice.

Many disabled people will not be able to wear the usual sort of clothing. Normal clothing should not, however, be constricting in any way and, if possible, the feet should be bare. It is quite all right to have a pair of thick socks which can be slipped on or off as required.

In our world we are always anxious for people to show us how to do things, but basically yoga is about inner understanding and so specific teaching should be kept to a minimum. Even with the postures, as the principles are learned, so the participant can devise his or her own programme and modifications. Always balance out activities and always finish up with a period of relaxation.

8.

THE ART OF RELAXATION

Aspects of relaxation have been discussed already, but the subject is one of such great importance that it merits a special section to itself.

As I have already emphasized, relaxation is one side of the coin of life. It is a counter-balance which makes our tension and our will-power effective. Some time ago it was realized medically that when human beings are subjected to a sudden challenge they automatically respond with a whole series of internal psychophysical changes which have become known as the 'Fight or Flight Syndrome'. As *homo sapiens* developed he had to be able to make an immediate and effective response to sudden opportunities and sudden danger. Generally these related either to the opportunity of getting food or to warding off a predator. Humans became adept at these responses and this adeptness has been partially responsible for the development and growth of our species while many others have died out or been subjugated.

'Fight or Flight' is merely the extreme of activation, an emergency series of changes to provide instant energy either for battle or for running away. We have discovered that, under extreme pressure, we can achieve things which we never believed possible. The 'Fight or Flight' aspect had been accepted for a number of years before it was clearly understood that the antithesis of these emergency changes was a process which has become known as the Relaxation Response. From this the realization has come that energization to a considerable degree depends upon relaxation. Disablement tends to heighten the tension aspect of life. Body tensions are created and not relieved; mental tensions are built up and not relieved. Many people diagnosed as having disabling illnesses say, 'Oh! I've got over that. I don't think about it now.' They are usually kidding themselves: what they mean is that they have swept the fear, the stress, under the carpet of the mind, pushing it into the subconscious.

A while ago a youngish woman with multiple sclerosis came to stay for a few days. I was just going away to an engagement but had a talk with her before I left. She told me she had come to terms with her illness and did not worry about it. Taking one good look at her, I said, 'I'm afraid you're a liar.' Then she admitted that every now and then the moment when she was told of the diagnosis suddenly came into her mind and she felt anxious and afraid and pushed it out again as quickly as possible. At those times her physical state got worse. I urged her not to let this fear creep up on her and weaken her, but deliberately to recall it to mind and to face it fairly and squarely. It would be very uncomfortable at first, but by doing this she would gradually exorcise the demon which was otherwise nibbling away at her, leading her to mental and physical deterioration. You cannot relax by dodging issues. Relaxation can only come from effective activation. This is a fact which is all too often ignored by those who profess to be teaching relaxation techniques.

Mental tension
The pressures of life today are creating thousands of stressed young executives, men and women. They become more and more bound up in themselves and their minds are full of anxiety. So dominating does this become that they give up other things to indulge their addiction of worry. They give up sport and activity; they give up hobbies; they give up much of their social life. Often they become convinced that they have a mental problem, that maybe they are going out of their mind and the obsession grows.

At first I simply tried to give such folk periods of

relaxation, but various tests showed that they were not relaxing and electronic tests usually showed a fixed, apparently degenerative state in the head. I began to think that perhaps they were right, maybe there was something wrong mentally. Then I had an idea. I got them to do something active before relaxing, sufficient to get their out-of-condition bodies panting heavily. Then I discovered that major changes could be detected and the head state quickly became much nearer normal. The reason was simple: the physical activity and the puffing stopped them from being so agitated about themselves and the brain quickly demonstrated this.

Disabled people come to this state all too easily because the condition of their bodies limits activity and encourages the wrong sort of 'going-in' on oneself. As I have already pointed out, the lungs are often largely full of stale air, the breath so shallow it can scarcely activate the brain and the heart is given no other stimulus than the none too healthy one of fear. To take such folk and tell them to relax is rather like taking a muzzled horse to the water and urging it to drink.

Naturally, I am not saying that at all stages of life it is necessary to do something active before relaxing, but where there is constant mental tension, combined with physical under-exertion, action is particularly important. Disabled folk cannot be asked to go out for a short jog, or even to jump up and down, so obviously other methods must be used. One of the simplest and most effective is the use of the Diaphragmatic Breath, already described. This is, in fact, more effective than many forms of physical exertion because it is controlled and uses the body correctly. Providing it is performed fully it will provide a wonderful basis for relaxation.

If required, where there is the capacity, a few rather more strenuous exercises than usual — and here I do mean exercises — can be undertaken. A higher pulse rate and better circulation will result and the brain can begin to enjoy the process of slowing down. At this stage it is important to discuss the differences between various techniques. We have simple relaxation (the 'sitting in a chair at home' variety) which is hardly relaxation at all. We have yoga relaxation, usually performed lying on the back, but quite possible in a chair if correctly understood, which makes one specific set of changes. We have visualization, which has already been described, and which makes somewhat different changes. Finally we have meditation, which is the deepest form of all. Meditation and prayer are terms which are often confused. One celebrated yoga swami defined the difference between the two as follows. He said: 'In prayer I am talking to God. In meditation God is talking to me.' However, meditation will form the subject of the next chapter.

Yoga relaxation
Having already discussed visualization, we are now concerned with the yoga form of relaxation. This can — and should — be practised on its own for periods of ten to fifteen minutes and it should form an integral part of any posture session, briefly between the postures, and at rather more length at the end. The physical requirements are as for visualization, but it is as well to go over them.

Firstly, for those sitting in a chair. The legs should be comfortable, firmly grounded and subject to minimum tension. The trunk should be upright. This is often difficult when sitting and certainly must not be rigid, but it is important to encourage this (the use of a pillow in the small of the back has already been advocated) and gradually to achieve it. A slumped person can neither relax nor meditate effectively. The hands should be joined on the lap and the head comfortably balanced on the shoulders, not falling forwards, backwards or sideways.

The eyes should be gently closed. For those lying on the back, the legs should be apart (a pillow placed between the knees if necessary), the ankles as loose as possible with the toes falling out. (Stiff legs and ankles will often respond to gentle help, which should be discontinued as soon as possible.) The arms need to be away from the sides, with the palms upwards (though not stiffly upwards). The back should be flat against the ground; here again a cushion (as small as possible) may be used for support if necessary.

The shoulders should be brought down (tension forces them forward) and the head kept in a straight line with the body. Where needed a small cushion may also be used here but the neck should be free — the chin neither pushing into the chest nor falling away. The eyes, of course, are closed. It is as well to experiment with these positions other than at relaxation time, because for many they are not easy and practice will be helpful.

It is important first of all to become aware of the breath and never to lose that awareness. Listening to the sound is helpful, feeling that it is not impaired, that it is slow, that it is rhythmical — that it is above all being enjoyed. Never forget that breath is life. Be aware of the gentle rise and fall of the abdomen, the relaxed stillness of the chest. Never be in a hurry; forget time.

Dispassionate observation
The core of relaxation is observation: first of the breath, then the body itself. One is a dispassionate observer, not activating anything, not fretting about anything. In this state of observation the body functions almost entirely autonomically. The breathing is not consciously directed — you are not breathing, the body is breathing. This does not mean that all body systems immediately begin to work rhythmically and in harmony. Far too many interruptions to the natural processes have taken place over the years and these interruptions have formed new, potentially or actually harmful, reflexes. In the state of true relaxation some of these reflexes will right themselves because of the easing of pressures which have normally operated. For example, skin circulation improves as one relaxes and the tensions are reduced. Many other aspects of daily bodily functioning are also improved. The improvements can come about only through observation and dispassion. At this stage one cannot try to make changes, only note the areas of tension or 'dis-rhythm' and let the brain/body make its own changes.

This form of relaxation is an essential aspect of life and we neglect it at our peril. The physical positioning which has been followed for centuries in yoga is one which diminishes physical tension to the greatest degree and therefore this process should be followed wherever and whenever possible. However, this is not always practicable even for the ambulant, let alone the chair-bound, and we can hardly argue that man is so designed that he must lie down carefully on his back every time he wishes to relax. (Incidentally, some people, especially those with back problems, may relax far better on their stomachs.) It is important, however, to remember the design of the human trunk. If we slouch or thrust our chest out we are not only throwing the spine off balance, we are also affecting the nervous system and throwing the back muscles out of their natural alignment. It is also important to reduce pressure on the abdominal area caused by slumping. So whether we are lying or sitting, having seen the posture is correct, we always pay attention to our breath next, feel it to be slow, rhythmical and free, with simply the abdominal movement. We then assume the role of *neutral* observer of the body. If some part feels tense, notice it calmly and without emotion. This very attention will diminish the trouble.

Many people use a relaxation process by which every part of the body is tensed hard and then relaxed, working from the toes to the top of the skull. This does have a little value but the real problem is not the tension in the areas themselves, but the mental process which is causing the tension. If the mind is concerned, worried or agitated, physical tension will return within seconds of any physical attempt at release.

By observing the body as calmly as possible we provide an initial impetus for the body to relax physically. The feeling of physical relaxation is a most satisfactory one, so this in turn enables the mind to let go a little. It is a mutually supportive process.

Relaxation is often practised with colourful imagery, sometimes sentimentally. This is not really helpful. Firstly, as with meditation, the relaxation process should be centre-pointed and not wide-ranging. The wider we roam in our thoughts the less we can induce mental calmness. Similarly, the whole point of relaxation is to maintain the observer role, inducing a mild state of heightened consciousness. We wish neither to lose awareness of the body nor to activate the body. This is what differentiates it from visualization. This is a positive and controlled mental stimulus to achieve a specific objective. Relaxation is the generalized letting-go of harmful disruption of body function, with resulting mental satisfaction.

It is important to understand this and not to allow confusion to set in. There are many relaxation tapes available, some of them excellent, but others do go into doubtful areas which are not central to the process of relaxation itself and it is important to be discriminating. If the tape does not conform to the principles I have outlined, then consider carefully whether it will really be of use to you. A similar consideration applies, of course, if attending a group where relaxation forms part of the programme.

Here is one specific approach to relaxation which can be memorized and used to advantage:

Lying or sitting peacefully but correctly, begin by paying calm attention to the breath and allowing it to settle into a rhythmical pattern. Do not rush this, especially if you have decided on the relaxation because you are feeling stressed. In due course begin to realize that you are observing your body as a living organism: the lungs expanding and contracting; the heart pumping; the blood circulating; the organs functioning. Consider the countless activities always proceeding within your physical body. Take time for this consciousness of your body to become really total.

Next, return to awareness of your breath and realize that this is what activates the whole of the body with which you are now one. Become more and more aware of the breath and its role. Again, take your time; do not rush.

The third stage is to consider the brain itself, realizing that the breath is supplying the energy which is activating the brain and this amazing instrument in the head is receiving hundreds of thousands of sensory impressions all the time; that it has locked within it a lifetime of memories — impossible to conceive the number; that it is issuing commands which affect every part of the body, stimulating and inhibiting.

Slowly we have built up the picture of the functioning of the physical 'us' but clearly this is not a self-sufficient unit, for who is this 'me' who is making the detailed observation? So we move slowly and calmly to consider the mind itself, realizing it is a mirror on which messages

— all too often sub-consciously selected — are flashed. But even this does not satisfy, for who directs the process which we call discrimination and does discrimination mean merely selecting a path from the signals of the brain? Finally we are forced to look beyond the brain and beyond the mind and sense the ultimate consciousness itself, which man has for centuries called the self, the soul, an aspect of God (whatever we may mean by that word).

Slowly working our way from observation of the physical body, through the brain and the mind, we reach a state which we cannot understand in human terms but which we know is wholly satisfying. It is the state which we call 'absorption', losing our own identity in something greater. Now truly we begin to feel at peace.

It is important not to break this slowly and carefully built up chain abruptly. The jolt will not be helpful. So we very slowly bring ourselves back to everyday consciousness, begin to move the body and to stretch, eventually slowly opening the eyes. When it is possible to achieve a relaxation in this or similar form, the mind will feel immensely calm and refreshed and the body will have benefited greatly.

9.

THE QUIET MIND

We have considered the process known as visualization and have just devoted a chapter to the art of relaxation. It is important that we also discuss the process called meditation. All three processes involve quietening the mind, yet, although many people express interest in relaxation and there is growing understanding of visualization, the concept of meditation still arouses some alarm and agitation. It is even attacked by a few people as being a process of opening up to the devil! This last view is more a comment on the state of the person making it than an intelligent criticism of meditation itself. I was once asked by a Christian minister what I made of the suggestion that meditation exposed the meditator to the influence of evil and I pointed out, simply as one part of the answer, the immense physiological improvements which have been shown to follow meditation, some of which have already been mentioned in this book. I suggested that the body would certainly not relax and function better if the mind was in the clutches of the devil — on the contrary some form of physical convulsion would surely follow. He took the point.

Whatever may be our personal conviction of the force of evil, the argument also falls down over a central point. The critics claim that the process of meditation is to make the mind blank and it is in this state that the devil may take over. However, it is made abundantly clear in yoga writings that it is quite impossible to make the mind blank

— this would, in fact, be death. The aim is to make the mind single-pointed; to be able to sustain a single, non-roaming, thought, with no urge to move away to anything else. It is interesting that the 'meditation and the devil' critics are almost always evangelical Christians, while eminent yogis in India often advocate that fixing one's mind on the vision of Jesus Christ is an admirable technique of meditation!

Since yoga regards man's path as the overcoming of suffering and meditation is central to yoga, it follows that meditation must be a powerful weapon to this end. At the beginning of this book I spoke of the miracle we have all performed by moving from an almost inert bundle to becoming able to use arms and legs fully. I pointed out that this was done without any instruction — it was intuition expressing itself. The second necessary miracle for man — learning to control the mind as we previously learned to control the body — is harder because we have learned language, which is a wonderful servant but a terrible master. Language has given us the 'I can't' syndrome, which is one of the most appalling psychophysical manifestations we have to overcome. So people spend a few minutes trying to be quiet mentally, find all sorts of stray thoughts crowd in and cry, 'I can't!' If we had known the dreaded words when we were babies we would never have walked. I am aware that I am repeating what I have already written but the lesson is a vital one.

Perseverance
If we really want to do something, we will persevere. As a youngster most of us want to ride a bicycle. We get on — and fall off. It happens time and again, but we have visual evidence that it can be done. We see others cycling around so we persevere until we achieve and then we never fully lose the art. A little older and the same process is repeated over car driving. Again, the stimulus is seeing others driving about and not wanting to be beaten. The difficulty about controlling the mind is that the result cannot be seen quite so plainly. But it does show itself in the life and the peace which ensues. Since mind and body are so inextricably interlinked it is obvious that the control of each

main component is essential for the effective functioning of the whole.

There is a very simple test which can be applied to confirm the mind's effect upon the body. Sit holding one arm out to the side at right angles, with the palm down. Ask a friend to place one hand on the shoulder of the limp arm and the other hand on the wrist of the arm which is extended. Now think of the happiest thing you can imagine, tense the muscles of the extended arm and ask your friend to try to push that arm back down to the side. It will be difficult, sometimes almost impossible. Now extend the arm once again, think the unhappiest thought you can muster and ask the friend to repeat the process. The arm will come to the side almost at a touch because, however hard you try, when you are unhappy you cannot tense the muscles effectively.

Think for a moment just what this means to the disabled person. The limb may already be weak: mental unhappiness will make it weaker. The person with a congenital disability often leads his or her life under mental tension, especially in the company of others who do not understand and accept the disability. As a result the whole body is further weakened. The person diagnosed as having a disabling disease suffers a major mental shock which is not eliminated, even though it may be swept under the carpet of the mind. Again, the whole body is further weakened. The single-pointedness of meditation is the process of stabilizing the mind with resulting mental strength, which then communicates itself to the whole body.

The deeper peace of meditation
How then do we achieve this? Firstly we must realize that the process of yoga is wholeness. Breathing naturally and effectively, moving the body naturally and effectively, relaxing naturally and effectively; all these are aspects of the same process and all lead to the deeper peace of meditation. For peace it is. Once the process of meditation has begun to 'bite' there is no turning back, for it brings a new dimension to life. Meditation, for the great majority of us, is the topping-up process of life. In a very real sense, all

life should be meditation, for we should retain the ability to be calm at all times and to sort through life, from the simplest chore to the most complex problem, with calmness and certainty. When we cry that we do not know what to do, which way to turn, we are actually saying that we are ourselves creating such a state of internal confusion that we 'can't even hear ourselves think'. One author has recently claimed that when we take up yoga we make the only necessary choice — to accept this way of life. After that there are no more choices because the calmness of yoga leads us to see what we need to do in any situation. To many of us that may seem to be a counsel of perfection but it is certainly a state on which we should set our sights.

The process, therefore, is as follows: first we re-educate ourselves to breathe naturally and well; secondly, we re-establish contact with our bodies; thirdly, we learn to counter-balance tension and reaction. The practical plan for such a process will be considered in the last chapter.

To many, meditation conjures up pictures of robed figures sitting motionless for hours on end in a most uncomfortable position. This is, in any case, a false picture and most of us can meditate effectively with quite modest requirements. Whether one sits on the ground, cross-legged or on one's heels, or sits in a chair, is not really material. What is important is that the back is erect. Some will find this difficult, even painful for a while, but as it is promoting the natural physical balance of the body it is important in its own right. While initially many disabled people (and not a few who are technically able-bodied) will be quite unable to sit erect, this must always be the aim and progress needs to be made towards it, however slow it may seem.

We must never overlook the damaging effects of torturing the trunk by bad posture and we must realize that these effects are mental, just as they are physical. The hands should be together in the lap, simply because this provides an energy circuit. Experiments, putting electrodes on the fingers, have shown how electricity leaks from the fingertips — on average about ten millivolts — and someone who meditates for a while leaving the 'circuit open' tends to feel uneasy and depleted. The head should be comfortably balanced on the shoulders and the great majority of people find it easiest to meditate with the eyes closed. There are schools of open-eyed meditation but, especially for novices, this tends to be distracting.

The first thing to realize is how intensely enjoyable true peace and quiet is. Most people will say how at peace they feel on a holiday when they lie on a quiet beach, on a still, sunny day and simply hear the gentle and regular lapping of the water on the sand. This is in essence a form of meditation. But we cannot spend our lives lying on peaceful beaches so, in one sense, meditation is a deliberate form of recreating such a situation, to bring about mental and physical peace.

Reference has already been made to a distinguished yoga swami who demonstrated at an American medical institute that he could slow down the pace of his heart remarkably, simply by sitting and meditating on a blue sky with small fluffy clouds which were hardly moving in it. He may have looked very mystical and esoteric, sitting cross-legged on the floor in his saffron robes with his eyes shut, but essentially he was doing the same thing as many of us have done while relaxing on a sandy beach — only no doctor has been on hand to check our heart beat! The difference is, of course, that the yogi is saying, 'I do not have to wait until the right time, the right place, the right temperature and the right state of mind come along; I will achieve the same results at any time and in any place.' In other words he is saying that he will control his own life, not leave it to the whim of circumstance.

In the happy holiday situation I have described, although we may not notice it, our breathing will be calm and regular — or get as nearly so as possible. When, therefore, we are taking our destiny and bringing it under our own control, we consciously see that the breathing is both calm and regular. Not by straining for effect, but by creating the thought of such a breathing pattern and letting the body follow the thought. If the thought is firm enough (but not tense) this will happen. Never doubt the power of your thought. So the first step is to take what is an end-product of the holiday peace and make it the first product of your mentally-controlled peace.

During the period in which the quiet breathing pattern is being established one should not try to evoke any special scene. The breath should be associated with a mood — one of warm contentment — rather than the surroundings evoking the mood. We know how we feel in those (often rare) moments when tensions drop off and all the world seems at peace. We also know that at such times we become less and less conscious of ourselves as individual human beings and merge in with the warm and peaceful surroundings. All this can be conveyed in the breath, with the attention only on the breath. Inevitably it will be slow, inevitably the out-breath will bring with it a physical sense of relaxation. Such single-pointedness over the breath can be maintained easily for two or three minutes, much longer as one progresses. The slow, calm sound of the breath is the soothing equivalent of the sea or any similar natural sound, into which we are able to let go.

In the early stages of meditation it is quite possible to do no more than to evoke a specific scene from the past which fits the contented mood of the breath, ensuring only that it is an essentially self-contained scene and one which does not set the mind roaming.

For example, it is quite useless to envisage the beach, to feel oneself lying there peacefully and then to see someone walking across the sand, recognizing the person and going with them in thought to some other place or incident. The beach must be free from anything which can allow the monkey-like mind to fly off at a tangent. If this peaceful vision can be maintained, with the breath providing the comforting natural basis of sound, we have already taken a first and valuable step towards meditation.

If such a vision is held, all told, for only ten minutes, it will be very helpful. Come out of it as you went in, allowing the scene to fade and for the last minute or so listening only to the peace of the breath. Then, slowly, open your eyes and have a little stretch. As simple a start as this will leave the mind feeling calmer, more positive and the body will be relaxed. Also, you will now want the experience to become a little deeper.

There are many good books on meditation and countless forms of meditation. Let no one try to tell you that theirs is the only way. So far as possible you need to find the form of meditation which suits you best. The repetition of a word or sentence is called mantra meditation. Some people use sacred words and phrases, others peaceful ones, still more say the words do not matter and it is the rhythm and feeling which counts.

I once knew someone who meditated for years very successfully on the sentence, 'Mary had a little lamb'! The mantra is repeated silently and again forms a single-pointedness of mood, rather than an intellectual analysis of the word or words.

I have mentioned that some yogis meditate on an image, such as that of Jesus Christ. This is an extremely effective form of meditation. It is also one which is a little wider-ranging. One chooses a figure with whom one feels deeply in sympathy. A contemporary example could be Mother Theresa, who is internationally known for her work for the poor in Calcutta. One would need to have seen a picture of her to conjure her up in that wonderful thing, the mind's eye. Inevitably she will seem calm and peacefully self-possessed and this will have a beneficial effect upon the meditator. Then it is permissible to consider in meditation the qualities which make such a person so different from her fellows: love, devotion to duty, tranquillity and so on. We may know that our own lives will never achieve a hundredth of the quality of such a person, yet admiring and understanding such a quality will affect us beneficially and also give us a true sense of humility.

A mantra which does conjure up a vivid picture and which I have used successfully in meditation, is the sentence: 'I cried because I had no shoes, until I met someone who had no feet.' This is not merely to remind ourselves of the suffering of others but of the fact that life endures despite suffering. Suffering, far from extinguishing the spark of life, often fans it into a flame. Then, in the deepest sense, the suffering is overcome. A process of meditation akin to that of visualizing a figure is that of taking a natural object. One commonly advocated is a rose: to see a rose, one single bloom and to be content to dwell on its beauty; to see every petal and the curve of the petals, the harmony of the whole, almost to smell the scent of the flower.

Slowly, but surely bringing the practice of meditation into one's life is slowly but surely to bring peace into one's life and to give the body the greatest opportunity of functioning naturally and well. I suggested that ten minutes would suffice to start with. This can slowly be extended. Some, who find themselves drawn to meditation, will in due course meditate for long periods. For most of us, half an hour is sufficient at any one time.

Showing a great understanding of psychology, classical yoga urges that meditation should be undertaken in the same place and at the same time each day. This is because the brain loves routines. Almost everyone knows of Pavlov's experiments in which he taught dogs to expect food at the ringing of a bell. In their anticipation of the food they automatically began to salivate. In due course he rang the bell, but did not provide the food. The dogs continued both to come to the sound of the bell and to salivate, even though no food was forthcoming. The mind of the meditator who can use the same place and the same time each day will calm itself in anticipation of what is to come, in the same way that Pavlov's dogs slobbered in anticipation of what they had been led to expect at a certain time. Such conditions are not, of course, essential but they do make the process easier. It will be possible to perform postures well and with calmness if the mind learns to say, 'This is when I do my exercises; it is all right; I can relax.'

It is an interesting fact that in the West in recent years the more physically active aspects of yoga have been embraced more widely by women than by men. On the other hand it is often men who express interest in meditation. As I have already explained, however, yoga has to be seen as a whole in which each aspect complements the rest and all aspects work towards controlling our mental activities, to bring us a true sense of peace and control, both over our lives and over our physical body.

10.

PUTTING IT INTO PRACTICE

Many books are written which give valuable advice and information. They read with interest, sometimes even with avidity; the reader feels in full agreement and vows to change. Then the book is finished, it is put on one side and all too often only an uneasy recollection remains. At the lowest level, I would not want you to waste the price of this book. Even more, I would not want you to lose sight of the changes which yoga can bring into your life. How can we best hope to achieve this? Firstly, let us review the basic facts:

(i)   The body is a living, self-repairing organism.

(ii)   The mind has immense power: for personal advancement or destruction.

(iii)   Body and mind work together, with the brain as the intermediary, in every aspect of life.

(iv)   Whatever may be the cause of disablement, the life of the disabled person will be in the hands of the body/mind.

(v)   There is a place for pills, injections, medical wisdom, operations, treatments etc. but they are all on the fringe and, at best, stimulate the body/mind process. At worst, they can harm or even kill. This must never be forgotten.

(vi)   The central fact is that our life is in our mind.

(vii) Our body, our brain, our mind are congruous parts of a wholly inter-linked system, the principle upon which the universe functions. How we see the words purpose, God, creator, is immaterial: they are all ways of looking at an integrated scheme of being, of which we are inextricably a part.

(viii) Being such a part we are directly linked to the strength of the whole — thus, whether we realize it or not, we are actually strong.

(ix) To use the means (the strength) to a right end (a good integrated life) is correct motivation.

(x) With correct motivation and constant renewal of our understanding, we can achieve.

Those are my ten principles of life. Never underestimate the strength of the conditioning we are under. It has been dinned into us ever since we were born, it has created a mass of reflex patterns of thought and behaviour which all too often make us feel trapped. But we are not trapped. We are surrounded by instances of people who have achieved wonders, because they found themselves on the right path and let nothing deflect them from walking that path. It is wise to study the lives of such people — not all of them famous, many nothing to do with religion or the so-called areas of 'do-gooding' — for this study can do much to strengthen our own resolve. Fundamentally, there is no difference between the greatest saint and the greatest sinner; the strongest person and the weakest. In every case the real 'us' is the same, only the façade is different. We can call on the real 'us' if we let ourselves do so, by working towards calmness and bringing a modicum of peaceful stillness into our lives.

To overcome the worst aspects of conditioning (remember that much conditioning is beneficial) we must establish our own discipline. Sadly, the word discipline has become an emotive one and conjures up a picture of something harsh and unpleasant; an uncomfortable process in which we are supposed to persist for the 'good of our soul'. If we understand yoga correctly, and seek to practise it correctly, the difference in the yoga concept of discipline soon becomes apparent. However strange it may seem to us, because of the lives we have led, yoga is a *natural* process. Yoga is life as it is designed to be, not as we have made it.

Posture

Let us just examine this at one simple level only: posture.
Over the ages man developed a unique design among the
creatures of the earth. He stood naturally erect, not merely
using erectnesss as an occasional alternative to going on
all-fours or some other position. This natural erectness has
become basic body design: the curves of the spine, the
positioning and tensioning of the groups of trunk muscles,
the functioning of the ribs, all are based on erect carriage.
A young child has it and uses it but as the world makes its
mark on that child, both physically and psychologically,
the posture changes and many a teenage youngster today
has round shoulders and a stoop, or else a defiant thrust
forward of the chest. These changes have been imposed on
a frame not designed to take them. As a result, to consider
one area only, we learn that around one-third of adults in
the West have back problems. Two extensive investi-
gations carried out in America showed that about eighty
per cent of the back problems were postural in origin.

I have mentioned that both physical and psychological
factors apply. Recently a young journalist came to see me,
sent by her doctor. She had realized that her bad posture
was bringing her neck and lower back pains and she
wanted advice on how to eliminate the difficulty. She
related it all to sitting over her typewriter and then, on
getting up, walking badly. What I soon discovered by
talking to her was that she also had a father who was an
alcoholic and she was continuously worried about money.
So if one considered the postural problem merely as a
physical one, the state of mental un-ease would always be
countering any attempts to get the posture right.
Unhappiness and worry have an immediate and
detrimental effect on the neuro-muscular system.

The discipline of yoga works upon both factors at one
and the same time. The physical movements correct the
wrong use of the body; the basis of the calm, natural
breath, promoting the calm mind, works at the same time
on the mental level, thus relieving the body of the burden
which worried thoughts impose on it. This is what I mean
by saying that the discipline of yoga is designed to bring us

back to the natural state. It is not a case of, 'My God! I hope this is doing me good because I feel terrible!' as with so many man-made disciplines. Practise yoga steadily, gently and calmly and it will become a natural addiction! Nothing is a greater stimulus to us than feeling better — without the possibility of side-effects.

What, then, must this discipline consist of? I can offer only the basics. The capacity of everyone is different, even the requirements can vary greatly. I urge you only not to under-sell yourself; realize you have more capacity than you believe and providing you are calm about it you can tap that capacity. Do not be determined with a capital 'D' — that is an unrelieved tension and it is ultimately destructive. Be quietly determined because you know you have the strength. I would urge you to remind yourself steadily of the ten principles which I have given at the beginning of this chapter. They are truths, they are common sense, but the pressure of a stress-ridden society all too easily erase them temporarily from our mind, changing 'I can' into 'I can't'.

Letting go of resentments
It is also vital each day to accept and to let go of resentments, frustrations, fears, anger. If you feel tempted to say you cannot do this, then throw this book away now. You are declaring that you are trapped within a negative mind and a negative body and you cannot get out. If that is the case, give up trying; do not waste your time, mine or anybody else's. If you face it as ruthlessly as that, you will realize that such an outlook is rubbish. You have just got yourself into a slough of lethargy, your breathing is terrible, your energy level is abysmal — but while there is breath in your body you can make the change. No one else can. Nobody can breathe for you; nobody can think for you. Every day should begin with an affirmation of life and of strength. Someone once said that the right way to start the day was by sitting up and crying. 'Good morning God!' If that sounds silly, reflect that the alternative is to sit up and say, 'Good God! Morning!' Many people seem to pride themselves on their sluggishness when they wake up. 'I'm no good for at least a couple of hours,' they say

smugly. Of course, our metabolisms differ, but consciously to face the new day with a positive affirmation is invaluable. One of the major difficulties which many disabled people face is that of purposelessness. Those who no longer work (or who have never been able to work), whose life drifts from day to day, have little incentive to wake up and perk up. Yet whenever such a person makes the change, many good things follow.

It is a central contention of yoga that we must change every downbeat negative thought into an up-tempo, positive one. This is an immense and daunting task, for most of us have thousands of negative thoughts every day. Yet it is not quite so difficult — even impossible — as it seems.

Reflexes
I have referred several times to reflexes. These in themselves are neither good nor bad. Within us are series of good reflexes, at the psychophysiological level — that is, calm brain messages incepting natural body reactions. The conditioning of life tampers with many of these reflexes, removing the natural and imposing an ineffectual or even destructive reflex in its place. So our task is to school ourselves back to having as many good reflexes as possible. Invaluable in assisting this process are memory reflexes: memories which pop up automatically, given the correct stimulus. Breathing is an excellent example here. Normally we think little about it, occasionally being half-aware that it is behaving oddly. When we begin regularly to improve the natural breath we register a much greater concern in the brain and, before long, the result is a strong reminder whenever our breathing gets 'out of sync', giving us the opportunity of putting it right again, with the inevitable resulting good effects.

The same process can apply when we determine to oust negative thinking. We will become more acutely aware that our thoughts *are* negative and that this is against the policy we have laid down for ourselves. Often this will result in some mental agonizing and for a while we will still complain to ourselves that we cannot change, but the spur is there and if an 'Improve your breath' reflex is

joined by an 'Improve your thinking' reflex, you know
very well that you have the power to make the change.
These daily processes of affirmation do, therefore, play a
very real part in our lives.

Whatever excuses we may make for getting out of other
aspects of the daily discipline, we have none which should
prevent us from consciously breathing better. Learning
how to breathe better and then practising it is no hardship;
it is a positive pleasure. This is the point which I must
emphasize yet again: because it is the very basis of life,
breathing is enjoyable; it should never be made a chore. In
trying to deepen and restore your natural breath be careful
never to strain. Let it happen slowly but surely and feel the
benefit as you practise.

I have taken care to show how we can work on and
restore our patterns of breath quite simply and without
any special preparation. The one essential is conscious
attention to it. Breathe fully for at least a few minutes when
you awake, thus removing mental and physical
sluggishness which often accompanies a night's sleep. Do
the same thing once more when you are up. During quiet
periods of the day remember that a little practice will pay
dividends. Study the relevant part of the book, keep it
handy and be sure that you have correctly understood the
basis.

The yoga *asanas*, or postures, combine the value of
enhancing the relationship between mind, breath and
body and the physiological (also mental) benefits of using
the body correctly. Unlike breathing, however, these
normally need more preparation and at least fifteen
minutes should be set on one side for the practice — more
if possible. Two sessions a day are really beneficial, one in
the morning and one in the evening. It will be seen that the
quite simple movements I have described can be
incorporated also into daily life. The stretching
movements, for example, can be practised at any time. The
important thing is that they should never become merely a
habit; they should also be practised with care and
attention, even if only as a brief interlude at any time,
sitting in chair or wheelchair. Relaxation is most commonly
practised as part of a session of movement but there is, of

course, no reason why it cannot be practised on its own.

When we come to visualization and meditation we need to be careful not to try to do too much. Generally speaking it is advisable to practise one or the other for a spell and not try to fit in both: it is quite possible to get yoga indigestion. Visualization is for a specific purpose; meditation is for the enhancement of our life. Wherever possible, it is sensible to try to keep a diary of progress. This is something which helps to keep us up to scratch, gives us the chance to sort ourselves out and enables us to look back from time to time to help establish the changes which have taken place, memory often being a very fickle thing.

*   *   *

Above all we need a sense of perspective. To see how tiny and unimportant is our own petty, individual life, is in no way to denigrate the importance of that life. It is a part of the whole and the whole can never be the whole without it. If you worked on a jigsaw puzzle which had one piece for every human being on this planet — more than four thousand million — and eventually, when you had almost finished it, you found you were one piece short, you could never claim to have completed the puzzle. Whether that missing piece was the largest or the smallest would be immaterial. Everything in life is integrated. That it appears to include injustices and accidents and tragedies only indicates our inability to see the whole pattern. Whether we are a king or a beggar, our part in the pattern is integral. Likewise, a play will have a variety of parts to offer actors. The big parts may seem the most attractive but the value of such a part may be wholly destroyed if, at the critical time, there is no one to come on and announce, 'Dinner is served.' Similarly — as Shakespeare himself noted — life is a form of play-acting. A poor actor does not work hard on his part and does not convince. A 'ham' actor becomes so totally involved in his part that he, too, does not convince. The great actor plays his part brilliantly and convincingly, by always keeping a tiny but very real gap between his performance and reality. At all times he is in command and in this lies his brilliance.

This, then, is the way we should look upon our individual lives. It is right that we should study our lives and lead them very fully; but at all times we need to be aware that the reality is something much greater than we can possibly realize and we are a part of that reality.

In recent years many people have come to realize that the disabled person should not be disadvantaged unfairly. Facilities are now improved, although there is still great room for further improvement. Such material considerations, however, must go hand in hand with mental ones. First of these is the realization that the disabled person has some physical limitations which are inconvenient, even distressing, but that is all. In some ways disablement is no more outlandish than baldness! Working for the sensible rights of the disabled person, therefore, must be linked with the understanding that disablement is only a word. There are no such groups as 'the disabled' or the 'able-bodied' — there are only people, and we should never forget that. Therefore I end by reminding all who read these words of the magnificent, and above all true, declaration of the Buddha:

Set your heart in one place
And nothing is impossible to you.

Appendix

WHEELCHAIRS

To suffer from physical disability is bad enough. To be pushed down in the name of help is even more concerning. Yet this is happening in far too many cases, with many people suffering both physically and mentally as a result.

The particular problem we are considering comes with those who have to take to a wheelchair more or less permanently. This in itself is a distressing thing which does no good to the morale of the affected person. If it really is essential (and many people are prematurely confined in this way when their ability to retain mobility has not been properly explored) then the resulting wheelchair, and the way it is used, should be designed to give the person the greatest possible help, not hindrance.

I had been feeling increasing concern about the difficulties posed by wheelchairs when, on a visit to Belfast, I was asked to visit a forty-six year old ex-nurse, who had been confined to a wheelchair for daily use for some considerable time. When I arrived she was slumped in her chair, looking tired and depressed. The ability to breathe well and rhythmically is essential in combating disablement but this woman's breathing was slight, with virtually no movement of the diaphragm. Trying to straighten her up, to give the ribs some chance of moving, I found to my horror that her back was now rigidly curved, with the shoulders in and the chest squeezed. This was no part of the disease, simply a seizing-up of the back from

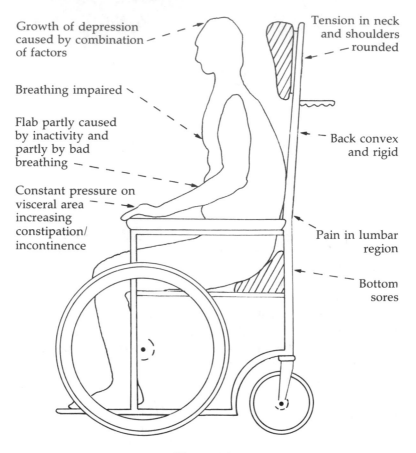

Growth of depression caused by combination of factors

Breathing impaired

Flab partly caused by inactivity and partly by bad breathing

Constant pressure on visceral area increasing constipation/ incontinence

Tension in neck and shoulders — rounded

Back convex and rigid

Pain in lumbar region

Bottom sores

Figure 26.

being in a constantly slumped position. The result was that she was fighting not merely disease but a whole range of other difficulties. They are shown in Figure 26. Her position had become more serious, but not yet permanent and within twenty minutes it was possible to begin to get her shoulders back, the chest slightly rising so the ribs could once again move and stretch the diaphragm. Even in that short time she began to feel a little better both physically and mentally.

It is important that the difficulties presented by wheel-chairs should be faced and overcome. The need for better-designed backs to the chairs is urgent (maybe some of the more expensive ones provide this, but models most in use only have a plastic or similar back which provides no proper support for the spine). While we are waiting for better chairs — and even after they are available — there are many things to be done which will not only brighten the life of the person concerned, but also improve his or her physical health and thus the resistance to the disease.

Compare the first picture with Figure 27. It is not suggested in the second picture that this position should be adopted all day, although it will become increasingly

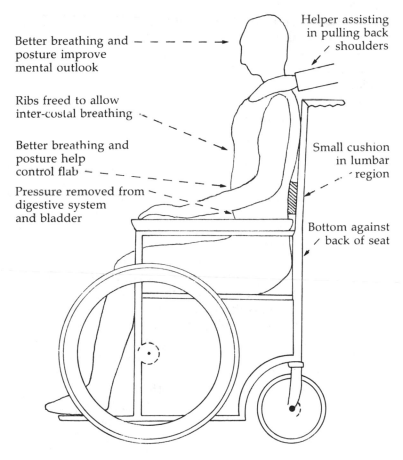

Better breathing and — — — — — → posture improve mental outlook

Helper assisting in pulling back / shoulders

Ribs freed to allow inter-costal breathing

Better breathing and posture help control flab

Small cushion in lumbar region

Pressure removed from digestive system and bladder

Bottom against / back of seat

Figure 27.

comfortable. At first this is to be adopted for a period of time, where possible with practical assistance from a helper. The first thing is to see that the person is helped to sit right back in the chair, with the bottom against the back of the seat. Many helpers allow the sufferer to slump into the chair, leaving the spine badly out of shape. This may just about be all right for us lazy people 'lounging' in an armchair for short periods, but we can straighten up at will as soon as the discomfort becomes apparent: the person with disablement often cannot. A small, reasonably stiff, cushion should be constructed, about five inches deep, to fit across the lumbar region, being tied by tapes to the back of the chair. Such a cushion could be made of high-density foam or a really compact stuffing. This will enable the spine to be held in the correct concave shape at this part of the back, with the resulting raising of the ribcage and chest.

The many benefits from such a posture are clearly shown in the drawing. Most important of all are the benefits to the breath, which can now be used to generate effective body energy. In the slumped position most of the breathing will inevitably be into the apexes of the lungs, with resulting disuse of much of the lungs and depletion of energy, physical and mental. In this position a helper can assist in the movement of the lower ribcage thus encouraging the diaphragm to stretch on the in-breath and relax on the out-breath. Sensitive but persistent pressure on the lower ribs on the out-breath will encourage the intercostal muscles to regain their elasticity and emphasis on the slowness of the out-breath will aid relaxation of the solar plexus area (with resulting mental relaxation), while removing much stale air from the lungs. Correct alignment of the shoulders can be assisted by the helper standing behind and working the shoulders gently back on the in-breath, allowing them to relax again on the out-breath. This again assists the shoulder muscles to resume effective action. Gentle movements of the head and neck will also help but these should always be carried out on the out-breath to ensure proper relaxation of the muscles.

Here is the sequence: keeping the shoulders still, breathe in and then, breathing out, slowly turn the head to the right. When the breath stops, stop the movement. Breathe in again without moving the head, allowing it to move further round again on the out-breath. The same thing can be done a third time until the head is turned to the greatest possible degree *without* pressure. Then, breathing in, the head is slowly turned to the front and, breathing out, to the left. The same process is adopted of moving the head only on the out-breath. Once again, breathing in, bring the head to the front, and, breathing out, let the chin drop on the chest. Now let each out-breath make the head feel heavier, so the back of the neck is stretched. After several breaths, bring the head up, breathing in and let it loll against the back of the neck. Clench the jaw and let it fall more heavily back with each out-breath, finally bring the head to an upright position once more. This form of head movement, using relaxation of the out-breath at all times, is excellent for removing the tension suffered by those in wheelchairs. Both breathing and mobility are assisted by raising the hands over the head slowly on the in-breath and lowering on the out-breath. This can be repeated several times. Leg movements can also be done to the same breathing pattern, according to the mobility of the

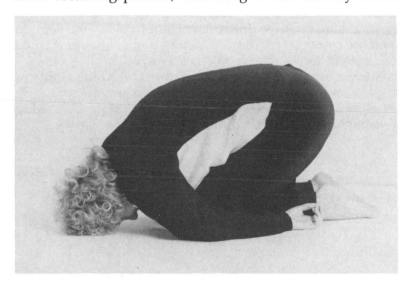

Figure 28. Pose of the child

legs. Where there is no apparent movement, the person should think movement into the leg on the in-breath: in certain circumstances this does, in due course, actually cause movement to occur.

Whenever possible those in wheelchairs should be got on to the floor, prone to their backs. This opens the chest and makes it easier to help with effective energizing breathing. Arm and leg movements can be organized from this position. In cases of spasticity, and often other forms of difficulty too, the Pose of the Child (or foetal position) can be extremely helpful. (See Figure 28.)

It should be remembered that however severe the problem there is generally more mobility in the body than is imagined. Once a real understanding of the breath has been achieved and the mind is quietened and aware (*not striving*), much can follow. The breath can also make a great difference in such movements as rising and sitting. Those in wheelchairs should always rise on a deep in-breath, even if they do not have mobility in the legs, and sit on an out-breath. The helper can stand behind the person, placing the arms under the armpits, beyond the point of the wrist. Pulling up sharply as the sufferer breathes in, will enable the person to rise with relative ease. Where there is insufficient strength in the legs to hold the standing position, a second helper should then be available to move the wheelchair away.

Human beings are amazing creatures, with the ability to inspire immense internal progress, if it is understood in the right way. Let's make sure that wheelchairs are used to help the sufferer — not to push them further down.

FURTHER READING

There are many books on yoga. Below are a few suggestions for those who would like to know more.

Barbara Brosnan, *Yoga for Handicapped People* (Souvenir Press 1982) (Primarily for yoga teachers and those working with the disabled, this is also helpful to the disabled person directly and is a splendid survey.)

Richard Hittleman, *Yoga for Health* (Hamlyn 1971) (The best known simple introduction. Very useful for those able to do a wider range of postures than those outlined in this book.)

Andre van Lysebeth, *Yoga Self-Taught* (Allen & Unwin 1978) (For those with reasonable physical ability. Comprehensive and detailed.)

Selvarajan Yesudian, *Yoga Week by Week* (Allen & Unwin 1979) (Also for the more active. Contains many helpful quotations and philosophical statements.)

Ramamurti Mishra, *Fundamentals of Yoga* (Lyrebird Press 1972) (For those who wish to study mental energization techniques more profoundly. From libraries only.)

Alistair Shearer and Peter Russell, *The Upanishads* (Harper & Row 1978) (Beautifully illustrated extracts from ancient texts with a clear translation. An insight into the original ancient wisdom.)

Howard Kent, *Day-by-Day Yoga*

Howard Kent, *My Fun with Yoga* (for children)

Howard Kent, *Key Facts: Yoga*

Tapes:

Howard Kent, *Yoga and Multiple Sclerosis* (Yoga for Health Foundation)

Howard Kent and Anita Ridges, *The Ickwell Experience* (Yoga for Health Foundation)

Howard Kent, *Deep Relaxation* (Yoga for Health Foundation)

INDEX